Practical Electricity in Medicine and Sur Liebig and George Henry Rohé

Publisher's Note

The book descriptions we ask booksellers to display prominently warn that this is an historic book with numerous typos or missing text; it is not indexed or illustrated.

The book was created using optical character recognition software. The software is 99 percent accurate if the book is in good condition. However, we do understand that even one percent can be an annoying number of typos! And sometimes all or part of a page may be missing from our copy of the book. Or the paper may be so discolored from age that it is difficult to read. We apologize and gratefully acknowledge Google's assistance.

After we re-typeset and design a book, the page numbers change so the old index and table of contents no longer work. Therefore, we may remove them; otherwise, please ignore them.

We carefully proof read any book that will sell enough copies to pay for the proof reader; unfortunately, most don't. Therefore, we try to let customers download a free copy of the original typo-free book. Simply enter the barcode number from the back cover of the paperback in the Free Book form at www.RareBooksClub.com.

You may also qualify for a free trial membership in our book club to download four books for free. Simply enter the barcode number from the back cover onto the membership form on our home page. The book club lets you access millions of books. Simply enter the title, author or subject onto the search form.

If you have any questions, could you please be so kind as to consult our Frequently Asked Questions page at www.RareBooksClub.com/faqs.cfm? You are also welcome to contact us there. General Books LLC™, Memphis, USA, 2012.

Assistant in Electricity, Johns Hopkins University; Lecturer on Medical Electricity, College of Physicians and Surgeons, Baltimore; Member of the American Institute of Electrical Engineers, etc.,

AND

Professor of Obstetrics and Hygiene, College of Physicians and Surgeons, Baltimore; Visiting Physician to Bay View and City Hospitals; Director of the Maryland Maternite; Associate Editor "Annual of the Universal Medical Sciences," etc.

PART III.

I. General Therapeutic Effects Of Electricity And

Methods Of Application,....251

II. Special Electro-therapeutics,....275

Appendix, 375

Index, 379

PREFACE.

It has been the endeavor of the authors to set forth, in the following pages, in a concise way, the fundamental principles which are involved in the application of electricity to medical and surgical practice.

The authors are well aware that the study of electricity presents many difficulties, and that to arrive at a practical knowledge of the subject (which is, without question, the knowledge demanded by the physician) whatever reading is undertaken should be supplemented by as much work as possible in the laboratory. The time required for an apprenticeship of this kind is, however, greater than the inclination, and, indeed, the duties, of the medical practitioner will permit. A treatise on medical electricity, therefore, to be of any value to the physician or the medical student, should be eminently practical, and should deal with such matters only as have a direct bearing upon the requirements of the practitioner. The book should be free from unnecessary technicalities, and only so much attention should be devoted to theory as is demanded in the explanation of such phenomena as are presented in the medical and surgical uses of electricity.

The subject of electro-static machines, of batteries (primary and secondary), of galvanometers, of various forms of resistance-coils (rheostats), etc., should be treated at length; while, on the theoretical side, the same thing should be done in regard to Ohm's and Kirchhoff's laws, to the best arrangement of cells in batteries, etc.

In the discussion of electro-static machines the laws of the mutual action of bodies in a state of electrification are necessarily involved, so that these laws must have been previously clearly presented, and the same is true in the explanation of the action of various other kinds of electrical apparatus. Hence, in order to understand the working of even the simplest forms of electrical appliances, considerable attention must be first devoted to the study of the elementary principles of electrical action.

These statements are made in view of a possible complaint that too much space has been given up to the discussion of electro-static machines. In further denial of the justice of "such a criticism, it may be stated that there is a very distinct correlation between the phenomena dealt with in electro-statics and those met with in magnetism and electro-magnetism. Hence it is that many phenomena have simply to be translated, as it were, from the language of electro-statics into the language of magnetism, the explanation remaining substantially the same. In consequence, time devoted to the study of one branch of the subject is so much time that can be saved in the study of the other.

The present volume has been divided into three parts, the first dealing with electricity and magnetism only, the second with electro-physiology and electro-diagnosis, and the third with the applications of electricity and magnetism to medical and surgical practice.

In Part I are discussed the various forms of electrical and magnetic apparatus likely to be of use to the physician in his daily experience with electricity, as well as the most suitable arrangement of cells for any given work, the construction and use of galvanometers, the theory of the chemical actions taking place in the storage-cell or accumulator, and the best methods of caring for such batteries.

A short description of the electric motor, the telephone, and phonograph is added, as all these appliances are continually, as time goes on, becoming of more value to the physician, either in the treatment or in the diagnosis of disease.

Part II takes up first the effects of electric currents upon the various tissues and organs of the body in health, then shows how these effects are modified by disease, and indicates the methods by which these modifications are utilized for purposes of diagnosis. A chapter follows descriptive of the various appliances most useful in electrotherapeutic work, which may be considered as immediately introductory to the section on electrotherapeutics.

In Part III the applications of electricity in the treatment of disease are considered. The methods by which electricity is made available for therapeutic purposes are described, and in subsequent chapters the modes of application of this agent in the treatment of the diseases of the various organs is indicated. Particular attention has been given to the applications of electricity in gynaecology, the diseases of the male genitourinary organs, and in diseases of the skin.

The illustrations in Part I are mostly original; of those in Parts II and III, Figs. 134, 135, 136, 164 and 165 are from Erb's "Elektrotherapie;" Figs. 138 to 163, from von Ziemssen's classical "Elektricitat in der Medicin;" 166 and 167, from Gowers' "Diseases of the Nervous System;" 168 and 234, from Lewandowski's "Elektrodiagnostik und Elektrotherapie;" and 222 from Dr. Ranney's work on "Nervous Diseases." Figs. 169 to 175 and Fig. 177 are taken from an article by Dr. Eoswell Park, in the "Annals of Surgery," and were reproduced by permission of the editor, Dr. L. S. Pilcher. The plates facing page 373 are reproduced from the "Atlas des Maladies de la Peau," of Prof. Sylva Araujo.

The authors have endeavored to place in the hands of the student and practitioner an intelligible account of the science of electricity, and a trustworthy guide to its applications in the practice of medicine and surgery. uWhether they have succeeded they now leave to the judgment of the reader.

Baltimore, January 1, 1890.

Part I.

Electricity And Magnetism.

Practical Electricity

IN

MEDICINE AND SURGERY.

CHAPTER I.

Electricity.

The groundwork upon which are based the modern theories of electricity and magnetism is, as in all physical sciences, an experimental one, and though theories may change from time to time, in accordance with increased and more accurate knowledge of the subject, the fundamental laws of electrical, and of magnetic actions as well, must always remain invariable. The laws have for the greater part resulted from careful investigations and well-directed experiments carried on in the laboratory and workshop, and are therefore completely independent of any hypotheses regarding the nature of electricity and of magnetism themselves. They remain the same whether there are two "electric fluids," or one electric fluid, or no fluid at all to be considered.

It is therefore quite unnecessary to attempt a definition of electricity or of magnetism, however desirable such a definition may be and however soon it may become a possibility. In the present state of science it is impossible to say what electricity is, but many of the laws which it obeys are well known, and a consideration of some of these laws and a description of such electrical phenomena as have a direct bearing upon the subject of medical electricity will be enough to attempt for the present.

By a common acceptation electricity has been called a fluid, and if we arc careful to remember that the term is used merely for convenience we shall not be led into error by adopting it in what follows.

Static Electricity.—The idea of two fluids has arisen from a consideration of the opposite properties exhibited by certain, bodies when rubbed together. When, for example, a piece of glass and a stick of resin, or a piece of ebonite (vulcanized India rubber) and a silk rag, are rubbed together and approached toward some small fragments of paper, the paper shreds will be seen to move under the action of the excited glass or vulcanite. The particles of paper will be attracted by the glass rod, and some will adhere to it for a few moments and then drop away.

The condition of the glass or vulcanite rod under these circumstances is referred to as *electrification,* and the agent which produces the observed effects is called *electricity*

If we should construct a sufficiently delicate apparatus for the purpose of testing the action, we should find that if the glass exerted an attractive influence the resin would exert an opposite influence, *i.e.,* it would repel. We should find in the same way that two pieces of glass which had been rubbed with resin would repel each other, that the two sticks of resin would act in a similar way, but that the glass and resin woidd mutually attract each other.

This shows us that the bodies—glass and resin—have acquired opposite properties, and, therefore, if we call the electrification of one of them *positive* we must call that of the other *negative,* though it is purely a matter of convention which particular state shall be positive and which negative.

In order to avoid confusion it has been decided to call the *Electricity at rest*—in equilibrium—is called static electricity. This we have to deal with in all eases in which bodies, having become electrified, are removed from the influence of disturbing causes.

Electricity in motion, i.e., electrification in its passage from one point to another, is called dynamical electricity.

In general, the two branches of study dependent upon these conditions of electrification are referred to as *electrostatics* and *electro-dynamics.* electrification of glass, when nibbed with resin, positive, or vitreous electrification" and that of resin negative, or resinous electrification.

Electrical Scale.—Many other bodies besides those mentioned are found to acquire similar properties when rubbed together, and by experiment it has been shown that, though one of the bodies is always positively electrified and one negatively, the sign itself is not determinate for any one body, but depends upon the substance by which it has been excited. Thus, in the case of glass it has been observed that, although when rubbed with resin it becomes positively electrified, when rubbed with the fur of a cat's skin it is negatively electrified.

In this way it has become possible to arrange a number of substances in a scale, such that a body taken at random in the scale will be negatively electrified when rubbed with «any substance which precedes it in the list, and positively when excited by any body following it.

  Cats' fur. Wood.
  Polished glass. Paper.
  Woolen articles. Silk.
  Leather. Shellac, etc.

Equal Quantities of Positive and Negative Electricity, and Value of Force Acting.—If we had been able, in the experiment just described, to determine the relation between the electricities on glass and resin, to measure also the value of the influence exerted by each body separately, we should have found that they were identical in absolute amount. We should have found that the *quantity of electricity* on the glass rod was exactly equal to the quantity on the stick of resin, though of opposite sign; that is,. the total electrification on any two bodies which have been rubbed together is zero, having due regard to signs. There are two methods of determining the value of the force exerted between two charged bodies. One method depends upon the fact first observed by Faraday, that there is no electrical force within a charged hollow metallic vessel, provided no charged bodies are placed »*cithin* it. Starting from this it can be shown that the force between two bodies charged with electricity is proportional to the square of the distance separating them.

The other method is to actually measure the force, as Coulomb did, with the aid of an apparatus known as a torsion balance (Fig. 1), though the method is not extremely accurate. Coulomb found, however, that, as a result of his investigation, the force exerted between two small spheres charged with electricity was proportional to the product of the charges—that is, the product of the quantities of electricity on each—divided by the square of the distance between their centres. If, for instance, we call the charge of one body E, and that of the other £", and place them at a distance apart equal to R, then the force between them, measured in certain units, is

„ $E\ E'$
$It3$

uWe can, therefore, double the force by doubling the quantity of electricity on one of the spheres or the other. Thus, if one sphere had a charge $2\ E$, the other having, as before, the charge E', the force would become $2\ E\ E'$

Tf, however, we had halved the distance between the centres of the small globes the force would have been $E\ E'$. $E\ E'$ or — («/2) R that is, four times as great as before. In the above examples we have supposed the bodies to have positive charges, and the forces measured would, therefore, be repulsive.

Conductors and Non-Conductors.—Let us go back for a moment toTthe fundamental experiment by which electricity was produced, of rubbing two bodies together; but, let us substitute a metal rod for the glass rod. Under these circumstances no electrification will be observed; even after the most violent friction the metal and silk will both apparently be unaffected. If. however, we had taken the precaution of fastening a glass handle to the metal rod, and had been careful not to touch the metal with the hand, a very sensible electrification would have been produced. The same phenomenon would have been observed, no matter what metal we had used, provided it had been attached beforehand to a rod of glass, resin, ebonite, sulphur, etc., etc. This shows us that there is a very marked difference in the ability possessed by bodies of keeping on themselves electrical charges. It shows us that the metals, though capable of frictional electrification, are not capable, under ordinary circumstances, of retaining a charge of electricity. It further shows us that the human body partakes somewhat of this property of metals, in that it allows electricity to pass through it. "We see, then, that bodies may be broadly divided into two groups,— those which retain electricity on themselves, and those which allow it to flow off. The latter are called Conductors, the former Non-conductors or Insulators. As in most classifications, however, so in this case, the distinction between the classes of bodies fades away at certain points. If we should arrange all known substances in the order of their conducting power we should find, at some place in the list thus formed, a number of substances which might be called indiscriminately either poor conductors or good insulators, just as in chemistry there are certain elements which strictly belong neither to the group of metals nor to the group of non-metals, and, in biology, living things which are neither of animal nor of vegetable origin, but are allied to both groups. For practical purposes, however, the line of separation is broad enough, and the following tables show with sufficient accuracy the order of a number of substances arranged according to their conducting or insulating power:—

CONDUCTORS.

1. All metals. fi. Metallic ores. 2. Chareoal. 7. Sea-water. 3. Plumbago. 8. Rain-water. 4. Dilute acids. 9. Living animals. 5. Saline solutions. 10. Flame, etc.

NON-CONDUCTORS.

1. Shellac. 10. Gutta-pereha. 2. Amber. 11. Silk. 3. Resins. 12. Marble. 4. Sulphur. 13. Camphor. 5. AVax. 14. Chalk. 6. Glass. 15. Lime. 7. Mica. 16. Oils. 8. Diamond. 17. Metallic oxides, etc. 9. Ebonite. *Induction.*—Let us observe the effect of suspending a glass rod, which has been rubbed with a silk handkerchief, within a hollow metallic vessel (Fig. 2), which completely surrounds it, the vessel itself being suspended by silk cords or supported by glass rods, i.e. , insulated. We shall now observe that the outside of the vessel has become charged with electricity of the same kind as that on the glass rod suspended within it, *i.e.,* positive, and that the inside has a charge equal and opposite to the external charge. If the glass rod be removed, no electrification can be observed on the vessel, inside or outside. This phenomenon, which takes place through empty space, is called *induction,* and the electrification of the vessel is said to be caused by induction.

The silk handkerchief being awkward for experiment, let us next rub a piece of resin with a glass rod and suspend first the glass rod within the vessel. If we move the glass around inside the metal case, always keeping it insulated and not allowing it to touch the sides of the vessel, we shall observe no difference in the charge outside, no matter whether the rod is near the metal sides or far away. Now bring the stick of resin also inside the vessel (Fig. 3); all signs of electrification will immediately disappear from the outside; which shows us that not only are the charges on the glass and resin of opposite sign, but that they are numerically equal.

Let us repeat the experiment, but now, before removing the glass rod from inside, let us connect the vessel by means of a copper wire with any very large metallic object, or even with the earth. Make a momentary contact, then break the con nection and keep the vessel insulated. The outside of the vessel will be without charge, but on removing the glass rod a negative charge will appear on its surface equal in amount to the former positive charge. The metallic object has received the latter charge, and it is said to have been electrified by ConDuction, its charge having been communicated to it through the copper wire.

A body is charged by conduction, then, when its electricity is conveyed to it through a metallic connection, and it is charged by induction when the electricity upon it is the result of the action of surrounding bodies, the action taking place through the intervening medium and at a distance.

It is usual to call the complete path through which the current flows from its source back again, the "electric circuit. " This may be composed of wires, of sheets of metal, of batteries, etc., etc., but the whole taken together forms the "circuit."

We noticed that when the sphere was discharged, the glass rod being suspended within it, another but opposite charge appeared on the surface when the glass was afterward removed. This shows us that when there are no charged bodies within the conductor its own charge is entirely on the surface. The same experiment furnishes us with the best proof that equal and opposite states of electrification are always produced at the same time. For if the glass rod had been more heavily charged than the resin the electrification on the outside of the surrounding vessel would have been positive, and if the resin had had the greater charge it would have been negative instead of being as it was,—zero.

Fig. *i.* Fig. 5.

Distribution of Electricity over the Surface of Conductors.—

If we charge an insulated conductor by induction, one end will have a positive charge and the other end a negative charge, the electricity being distributed in greater quantity (per unit area) at the nearest and most distant points, relatively to the inducing body (Fig. 4). At spme point *(B)* between the ends there will be no electrification whatever. In the figure, *A* is the inducing body, supposed to be positively charged, and *B* is the insulated metal rod. The distribution of electricity under these circumstances will be something like that shown in Fig. 5, in which the shaded portion about the rod represents the Active layer of electricity., *Faraday's Views, and Lines of Force.*—We may regard the phenomena of induction and of electrical attraction and repulsion in either of two ways: "We may suppose them the result of a direct action at a distance, or we may suppose that the influence is exerted between contiguous molecules of the surrounding medium. In the latter case the medium plays a very important part. Both views are held, but the latter far more generally at present than the former; and it is undoubtedly better adapted to the explanation—without the use of mathematical symbols—of the various problems we shall have presented to us. Faraday, in his exhaustive work in electricity, was the first to recognize the importance to be attached to the medium in transmitting electrical actions from one body to another, and he pictured to himself the state of the medium while these actions were going on. He supposed that the medium about a charged body was in a state of stress, and he represented to himself the forces acting, not as mere directions, but as a series of lines which continually endeavored to shorten themselves, just as India-rubber bands would do. These lines he called " *lines of force"* and the region around a charged body the "*electric field."*

According to this view, every charged body radiates out from itself into space lines of force, and every line shows at any point the direction in which a very small body would move if freely suspended at that point. These lines of force have their origin at the surface of the charged body, to which, if the body is a conductor, they are—at the surface—perpendicular. Where they end electricity of the opposite kind will be found, and the total amount, no matter how scattered it may be, will equal in value the charge on the original body. Part of the induced charge may be on the walls of the room, some of it may be on surrounding conductors, but, taken altogether, the total amount will be the same.

A few cases in which the lines of force around a charged body or bodies are known are given in the accompanying figures.

The simplest case is that of a sphere suspended at a distance from other bodies in the air (Fig. 6). Owing to the perfect symmetry of the figure the lines of force are radii from the sphere outward, and they extend away from the surface to an indefinite distance in straight lines. Another very simple case is that of a sphere suspended within a spherical shell which completely surrounds it (Fig. 7). Here the lines of force are also radii between the surfaces, and if we suppose the outer shell connected with the earth there will be no lines of force around it; that is, outside. Hence, all the force is in the intermediate space between the sphere and shell, and there is no force outside. If the interior body, instead of being a sphere, were also a hollow shell, there would be no force in the medium inside this. Another example is that of two spheres whose charges are in the relation of four to one and of opposite sign (Fig. 8). If both charges are of the same sign the lines of force assume the form given in Fig. 9.

If we knew the number and direction of the lines of force at any point due to charged bodies near it, we would have a solution of a very important class of electrical problems. It is, however, only in a very few cases that we know this, and the calculations necessary, in even the simplest cases, are very elaborate. Often, however, we can form some idea of the state of the surrounding medium, and by drawing, even roughly, the Figs. 8 and 9 are taken from Maxwell, "Elec. and Mag.," vol. i.

lines of force, we can obtain solutions of a few cases accurately enough, and thus accomplish in a few minutes what might require laborious work if undertaken by mathematics alone. The conception of lines of force is extremely useful, and we shall see more and more clearly, as we take up the study of magnetism and electro-magnetism, how easily certain phenomena can be explained by their aid. *Potential.*—We have now to take account of an idea that is of the utmost importance in the explanation of electrical phenomena; that is, the idea of *potential*. The conception has always been considered a difficult one in the study of electricity, though there seems to be no valid reason for this. At all events, it is absolutely necessary to become acquainted with the subject, for many problems cannot be understood at all without introducing the idea. The potential at a point near a body may be defined in either of two ways: We may define it as the charge on the body divided by the distance between the body and the point, or, we may define it as the work which would have to be done on a unit of positive electricity in bringing it from an infinite distance to the point in question. The former definition follows at once from the latter, which is therefore the more general and the more preferable.

Potential, therefore, is work done, and can be expressed in units of work, or, if we use the so-called absolute system of units, to be hereafter described, we can express potential, or differences of potential, in centimetres—grammes.

We spoke of determining the potential at a point by bringing from a distance a sphere charged with a unit quantity of electricity to this point. Here we must be careful to employ a very small sphere, since this itself, when charged, alters the potential at points near it. It would therefore exert a disturbing influence if the charge upon it were comparable to that of the body to which the potential was due.

Starting with the small sphere, having a unit quantity of electricity at a great distance from charged bodies, very little force will be required to move it. Now, suppose the charges are all positive; then whatever electrical force is exerted will be repulsive. As we move the small sphere nearer and nearer to the charged bodies the repulsion increases, and more force must be exerted in the movement; consequently, more work must be done, and, according to the definition given above, the potential must increase as we approach the charged bodies. Hence, at great distances, where the force is small and little work is done, the potential is low; whereas, in proximity to the charges, the force is great, much more work must be done to move the sphere from one position to another nearer the charges, and the potential is high.

It follows at once from the foregoing definition that bodies always tend to move from places where the potential is high to places where it is low.

The potential of a body being a relative thing, it is necessary to have some standard of reference, and the standard usually taken is that of the earth, whose potential is assumed to be zero. Sometimes, but as a mere conception, an infinitely distant point is taken as the point of reference, since at an infinite distance away from charged bodies the potential must be zero. This is, however, done for the sake of simplifying mathematical calculations only.

Electro-motive force is that which tends to set electricity in motion, or we can say that the electro-motive force (written *e.m.f.*) between two points is the difference of their potential.

Hence, when two charged metallic bodies at different potentials are connected by a conductor there will be a transfer of electricity from the one at higher potential to the one at lower potential, and the transfer will continue as long as there exists any difference in the potentials of the bodies.

Current.—This passage of electricity along a body is called the electric *current*. The phenomenon may be of short duration; it may last only the millionth of a second, but while the transfer is actually taking place there is an electric current in the conductor.

We must here be careful to distinguish between the electromotive force between two charged bodies and the mechanical force acting from one to the other. Electro-motive force simply urges electricity onward, and its amount is greater the greater the difference of potential. Mechanical force tends to bring the bodies nearer together or to drive them further apart, and we already have found how to measure it.

Equipotential Surfaces.—It is a matter Fig 10 of familiar observation that the electricity upon any charged body, whether conductor or non-conductor, but removed from electrical influence, is at rest. In other words, we know that the electricity upon its surface, under these circumstances, is in equilibrium. But, from what has been said, it is apparent that electricity will move upon the surface of a conductor, if between any two points on it there exists a difference of potential. Therefore the surface of the conductor must be everywhere at the same potential, and it is on this account called an equipotential surface. But there are other points about a charged conductor which have also among themselves the same potential, and the surfaces drawn through these points will be equipotential surfaces. The potential of each surface becomes less as we go outward from the charged body (Fig. 10), until at a very great distance the potential of the corresponding surface may be taken as zero. Fig. 10 shows the equipotential surfaces around a charged metal sphere, the sphere being supposed at a distance from other charged bodies. It will be seen that each of these surfaces is spherical, *i.e.*, a circle, in projection. Since the equipotential surfaces are spherical and the lines of force about a charged sphere are radii, it follows that the equipotential surfaces and lines of force are perpendicular to each other.

Many other cases might be given in illustration of the statements here made, but as we shall have to deal with the same subject more thoroughly in the study of magnetism the consideration of the matter may conveniently be deferred.

Potential Energy.—If we charge a body placed in such a part of the electric field that its potential is V, say, with E units of electricity, the potential energy of the body will be $E V$; for the potential V means the work which would have to be done on a unit charge in bringing it from a place where the potential is zero to the point in question. If we carry E units instead of a single unit, the work done will, of course, be E times as great, but, since the potential varies from 0 (zero) to V during the movement of the charge E, we must take the average value of the potential between 0 and V. This is J, so that we have for the whole work done— that is, for the energy of the charge—£ $E V$.

A very similar expression holds in the case of electric currents, and we shall find the formula of considerable importance as we go on.

Capacity.—Suppose we have two charged metallic disks, supported by non-conductors in such a way that the disks are parallel to one another, and separated by a certain distance which we will call D. If we connect the two plates with an instrument capable of measuring differences of potential we shall observe a certain value for this which we will call V.

Let now—the plates being still insulated—the distance between them be diminished, so that it becomes §; we shall find that their difference of potential will diminish also. In order to make the difference of potential the same as it was before the plates were brought nearer together we shall have to increase the charges correspondingly. If the distance between the plates had been halved the charges would have to be approximately doubled. This is expressed by saying that under these circumstances the Capacity of the arrangement has been about doubled. We define the capacity of such a system of plates as the quantity of electricity necessary to charge the plates to unit difference of potential, or, the potential of one plate being 1, of the other $V2$, and the charge on one of them E, then

Capacity =.

If, instead of moving the plates— which are supposed to be in air—nearer together, we had inserted between them a sheet of shellac or of vulcanite, an effect of the same kind would have been observed; that is, the capacity would have been increased by so doing.

Specific Inductive Capacity.—To this quality,—namely, of diminishing the potential between two bodies, their charges remaining the same,—possessed by a large number of substances in various degrees, that is, by glass, spermaceti, resin, pitch, wax, shellac, sulphur, etc., Faraday gave the name of specific inductive capacity, and the medium itself he called a dielectric medium. It is very different for different bodies. Thus, calling the specific inductive capacity of air unity, then, Faraday found that for wax it was 1.86 and for sulphur 2.24. *Condensers.*—An apparatus, consisting of two parallel plates (Fig. 11) or of a hollow conductor inclosing within itself another conductor, the two being separated by air or other dielectric medium, is called a condenser. Condensers of this form have a very limited range of usefulness in practice because their capacity is small; but standards are made in this way, and the most accurate form of instrument is that of a sphere suspended within a concentric spherical shell. The capacity of such condensers can be calculated at once when their dimensions are known, and others, of forms rendering calculation impossible, but more convenient for general work, can be compared with these and standardized. In the ca-R in which we have a ine lium other than air between the plates of the apparatus referred to we have to write for the capacity $C= E K$ being the specific inductive capacity, the remaining letters as before.

In the-construction of condensers it is usual to employ a large number of plates and to separate them by very small intervals. Generally, plates of tin-foil are used, these being separated by very thin sheets of prepared paper or mica, and several hundred of them placed together in a box. In this way the capacity can be made as great as we please.

Leyden Jars.—But the best-known type of condenser is the so-called Leyden jar (Figs. 12 and 13), which consists simply of a glass jar covered inside and outside, except near the neck, with tin-foil. On top of the jar is a brass knob in metallic communication with the inside coating, but insulated from the outside metal by means of a wooden stopper, through which the knob passes. Such a condenser, when made with thin glass, may have a very great capacity, and is altogether a convenient form for general work in electricity. There is danger, however, that, when the glass is very thin, it may be ruptured by the passage of a spark between the coatings, if they should be electrified to great differences of potential. This alone, however, is not the only circumstance which limits the difference of poten

Figs. 12 And 13.—Leyden Jars. tial which can be maintained between the outside and inside of the jar; it is also limited by the leakage which takes place between the inside and outside tin-foil over the surface of the glass. Glass, though usually an insulator, conducts fairly well in damp weather, when the electro-motive force is very great.

When we have to employ very high electro-motive forces, we join a number of Leyden jars together by connecting the inside coating of one with the outside of the other. This arrangement is known as the arrangement in series or in "cascade." Fig. 14 represents a number of Leyden jars connected up in this way. As will be seen, the first jar has its inner coating connected through the knob and wire with the outer coating of jar No. 2, which in turn has its inner coating in metallic communication with the outer coating of jar No. 3, and so on. The inner surface of the last jar is connected by a wire with the knob A, as shown, the knob B being connected with the outer coating of jar No. 1.

By such an arrangement the capacity of the jars, taken together, is less than the capacity of a single jar in the ratio of the number of jars; the difference of potential has,, however, become n times as great, supposing that there were / jars. This is not rigorously true, for the connecting wires have some capacity, but it is very small compared with the capacity of the jar itself.

Instead of joining up the jars in this way we may connect all the similar coatings together; that is, all the inside coatings with one wire, and all the outside coatings with another, as in Fig. 15. Such an arrangement is called the "quantity " arrangement, but it is better to say that the jars are joined in " parallel arc." In this way the jars taken together act as one very large jar, for if all the inside coatings are joined together the same effect is produced as if a single jar had a coating of tin-foil as large as the sum of the separate ones, the same being true for the outside. Hence, the capacity, if there are n jars, has been increased u times; but the difference of potential has remained the same as before. We may also express this by saying that to charge n jars joined in parallel requires n times the quantity of electricity necessary to charge one jar.

Finally, we may arrange the jars combinationally according to both methods, as in Fig. 16. In this case two jars form a set equal to one jar of twice the capacity, and the sets of two being joined in series give a difference of potential equal to twice that of a single jar. Many combinations can of course be made in this way, and the particular arrangement to be adopted depends upon the special work we may have in hand.

We can explain the theory of the Leyden jar very much better by taking for discussion a more symmetrical form of condenser than this.

We have seen that if we suspend a charged body 'within a hollow metal conductor (Fig. 17), the inner surface of the conductor in question will receive an opposite charge 'of electricity equal in amount to that on the suspended body. Now, suppose we have two spherical bodies suspended one within the other (Fig. 18). Since the bodies are perfectly symmetrical the charges must be evenly distributed over the surfaces, and the lines of force in the space between the shell and sphere will, as pre viously shown, be radii to the two surfaces. Now, to say that the distribution is perfectly regular is as much as to say that each unit of surface contains a quantity of electricity which we may call B; B is generally called the "electric surface density." But, the inner surface having a radius II, its area is $4 1 B2$, and hence, if its total charge is E, then $E = 7l It3 B$. Again, since we have the same quantity, but of opposite sign, on the inner surface of the surrounding shell we have also

— $E = 4 7t R3 Bl$ where R is the radius of the shell.

We have shown that the electrilication on the exterior of the shell is independent of the position of the influencing hotly within it, provided only the charge on the latter remains always the same. Furthermore, the direction of the lines of force in the intermediate space continues to be % along the radii to the spheres, both having the same centre, whatever size the internal surface may have.

Let us suppose, then, that the outer shell becomes indefinitely large, and that the inner one becomes smaller and smaller, so that it may finally be considered a point. The external effect remaining always the same, we observe that, instead of considering the charge over a sphere, we may replace this by an equal charge supposed at the centre of the sphere; that is, at a point. It follows, therefore, that the potential at any point outside a charged spherical surface is , where E is the charge and R the distance between the *point* and *centre* of sphere. At the surface of the sphere itself this distance becomes the radius of the sphere, hence the potential of a sphere due to its own charge is -, A being its radius.

According to the definition given above, the capacity of any system of bodies is the charge necessary to produce unit difference of potential. Hence, the capacity of a sphere, in open space,being its charge E divided by its potential , is A; that is, the capacity of a sphere is numerically equal to its radius.

We have shown that there is no electric force within a charged metallic conductor provided there are no charges inside; hence it follows that the potential must be everywhere the same inside such a body. Now, the potential at any point of the interspace between two concentric spherical shells (Fig. 19), whose charges are respectively --E and —E, and whose radii are A and B, due to the inner shell, is , and that due to the outer is

— . The potential due to both is then Fig.18.

For a point on the surface of the inner shell, or within this as well, R becomes equal to the radius, A, and therefore the potential becomes

M Bl

'which shows us that the capacity becomes greater the more nearly equal are A and B; that is, the more the two surfaces approach each other in size. The Leyden jar may be regarded as a particular case of the problem just considered, in which the air-space between the shells is replaced by glass, the shells themselves playing the same part as the tin-foil in the Leyden jar. It is therefore evident that the capacity of the jar is increased by bringing the tin-foil surfaces near together, *i.e.*, by making tbe glass as thin as possible.

Fig. 20.—Electro-static Machine. *Electro-static machines* may be divided into two classes,— those in which the production of electricity depends upon the friction between two surfaces, called *frictional machines,* and those in which the charge is the direct result of induction, called *influence* or *induction machines.* The latter usually have to be independently charged at first before they will act properly.

The theory of both classes of machines is uncomplicated after the fundamental laws of static electricity have been understood, but especially is this true of the former class. Indeed, frictional machines require nothing more for their explanation than an understanding of the phenomenon resulting from rubbing a piece of glass with silk or flannel.

Frictional Machines.—In its usual form the frictional machine (Fig. 21) consists of a circular glass plate *(A)* capable of revolution about its centre and provided with a "rubber" *(B)* and a metal comb (*C)*. The rubber is a piece of leather, having on one side an amalgam made of tin and mercury, this surface being in contact, under slight pressure, with the revolving glass plate. The comb is a rod of metal—generally brass—with numerous sharp points attached, which approach very near to, but do not touch, the glass disk. The leather and comb

Fig. 21.—Frictional Electric Machine.

are connected by means of wires or metal rods with a pair of brass balls, sometimes called the "prime conductors," but better known as the poles or electrodes of the apparatus.

The action of the machine is as follows: When a certain portion of the glass disk passes beneath the "rubber " it becomes positively electrified and the leather negatively. This positive electrification, or charge, carried around with the plate, in approaching the metal comb induces upon it an equal negative charge, while the positive charge passes toward the pole Dx in metallic connection with the comb. As the charged portion of the plate approaches still nearer the comb the difference of potential at last becomes so great that the comb discharges itself against the plate, thus annulling the charge on the latter, which passes again under the amalgam in a neutral condition. The discharge upon the disk is facilitated by the points of the comb, which are employed for that purpose.

In reality, all of the half surface of the plate acts inductively, but with varying intensity, upon the comb at any one time; but we have considered only a small part of the disk for the sake of simplicity.

It may be added that the discharge between the comb and the disk takes place in what is known as the brash discharge, which is a species of electric spray.

The rubber, which, on account of the amalgam, is a good conductor, transmits its negative charge to the pole $D2$ and the two poles having thus their charges continually augmented acquire finally such a difference of potential that a spark passes between them. The length of spark which can be obtained from such a machine is limited by the leakage which takes place over the glass disk between its own charge and that of the rubber. To reduce this as much as possible a flap of oiled silk is often suspended close to that portion of the plate which is electrified, *i.e.,* the upper half. When the difference of potential or electro-motive force between two bodies becomes very high the electricity flows from one to the other through the insulating medium in the form of a spark. Different media resist such discharges in different decrees, but any medium can be ruptured by a sufficiently high electro-motive force. The insulating power of air is comparatively great, but it can resist what may he called electric pressure only within certain limits, after which it gives way, and the electric spark passes, accompanied by noise and light. If the pressure is not so great as to produce sparks, and the electricity is distributed over points or sharp edges, it leaks away, in the form of a "brush or spray." and the phenomenon of the "electric glow" can be made very apparent in a darkened room.

Influence Machines.—Of the class induction or influence machines, perhaps the best known is the Holtz machine (Fig. 22), the essential features of which are shown in the accompanying sketches (Figs. 23 and 24). In its simplest form the apparatus consists of two varnished glass disks (4 and *B),* one of which (. 4) is stationary, the other *(B)* revolves about its centre. The stationary plate (. 4) has two openings cut into it *(Bu B2),* through which and toward the revolving plate extend a

B A pair of paper strips with pointed ends, marked Cx and C2. These are the prolongations of two pieces of paper, fastened to the plate just above the openings, and called the "inductors" (Z and *D2).* Opposite the inductors, on the other side of the revolving plate, arc a pair of metal combs (i *F2)* joined by wires with the poles of the machine, shown as Px and P_z Fig. 24.

The action of the machine may be explained in the following way: Let one of the inductors be charged,—say positively.— and let the two electrodes be brought into contact. As a result, the comb opposite this inductor is charged negatively by induction, and a positive charge appears at the other comb, since the combs are in communication through the joined electrodes and the positive electricity is repelled away from the inductor itself.

Since the combs consist of sharp points the negative electricity upon the first comb begins to discharge itself against the glass plate in front of it in the form of a brush. This negative charge is carried around by the plate in a direction toward the other inductor and comb. Both of these, therefore, discharge positive electricity on the plate,—the comb upon one side, the inductor on the other,—while the inductor itself receives a negative charge. Clearly, therefore, part of the negative charge upon the front of the plate is neutralized, and the positive charge upon the back is carried around again toward the positive inductor. This increases the action of the positive inductor, since the inductor itself discharges negative electricity upon the plate and becomes /" / itself more and more strongly electrified (+ ' f — 1 positively. If the electrodes are now separated, sparks will pass between them. The object of having the holes in the stationary plate is to diminish the capacity of those parts of the plate Fig.e. which are opposite them, and thus cause them the more readily to give up some of their charge. In some cases Leyden jars are attached to the electrodes, the object being to increase the energy of the sparks given off.

Current—To the passage of electricity through a conductor has been given the name of electric current, and in this sense the discharge of a Leyden jar is as true a current as is the movement of electricity in the wires which feed our electric lights and motors. There is, however, a broader sense still in which the term electric current may be used: we may understand it to mean any transference of electricity from one body to another. Tims, if we move, or rather, under the circumstances, allow to move, a very small body, an insulated metal sphere, between two electrified spheres (Fig. 25), we have, as long as the motion continues, the phenomenon of an electric current between the globes; that is to say, the small sphere carries electricity from one sphere to the other, and as long as any charge remains the little ball will keep up its motion, vibrating backward and forward. Such a current may be called a *convection current,* in contradistinction to ordinary or *conduction currents,* and it has been shown experimentally that if the velocity of a statically charged body be great enough it will exert an action altogether similar to that exerted by an ordinary current in a wire. We shall, however, for the present confine our attention to such currents as are furnished by ordinary batteries and dvnamos.

1 a 3 4-S 6 *l* 8 9 10. II
Fig. 28.

At this point it may be well to draw attention to the absurdity of statements sometimes made regarding the " quality" of electric currents. It is often averred that currents have various "qualities," the idea intended to be conveyed evidently being that electric currents have something of the character which distinguishes the notes of different musical instruments. This is, of course, absolutely ridiculous, the only character which currents, derived from whatever source, can possibly have—if we can properly speak of character at all in this connection—being fully included under one or another of the following heads. We can have:— 1. Steady currents.

2. Interrupted currents. 3. Alternating currents. *Steady Currents.*—Steady currents are usually furnished by cells of ordinarv type and by storage batteries, and we may represent them in this way: Let us use the vertical line (Fig. 26) to represent the value of the current measured in any arbitrary units (by means of a galvanometer, voltameter, or whatever measuring instrument we decide to employ). Let the horizontal base-line represent equal intervals of time,—minutes, or hours, etc. Then the horizontal line *A,* drawn through the figure 4, shows us that the current has the same value at the end of time 4 as at time 1, 2, and 3,—in other words, that it has not varied. Such a current, *besides being a steady one,* is a *constant current.* There are, however, few batteries which will furnish such currents during any considerable time, and generally the current continually becomes smaller and smaller, as shown in the lower dotted line *(B),* which, as it slants downward, indicates how regularly the current diminishes. The upper dotted line (C) represents the current derivable from a storage battery, in which there is a rapid decrease during the beginning of the time (that is, if the current is rather strong), alter which the current becomes *constant,* and remains so until the battery has become nearly discharged, when it falls to zero very rapidly. All these currents are steady. *Intermittent Currents.* —Of a different kind is the current supplied by an ordinary dynamo machine. In this case the current is not absolutely steady,—though for practical purposes it may be so considered,—but varies between certain limits many times during one second. This is due to one of the necessities of dynamo construction, and arises from the fact that the " armature" of such machines consists of a number of separate coils of wire in which the current is periodically reversed twice in each revolution. In general, however, the number of these coils is so large and the speed so high, and the effect is, moreover, so strongly modified by other actions going on in the armature, that the " waviness" of the current is not easily detected, though it is at once observable by means of a telephone. With the same notation as before, the dynamo current may be represented as in Fig. 27. Here, as will be seen, the current is subject to periodical fluctuations of intensity, and reaches maxima and minima values a certain number of times within a given interval. In the upper curve the fluctuations are more marked than in the lower one, but in all such cases, when we speak of the intensity of the current, we mean the average intensity; and, practically, the variations from the mean value are so small that we may entirely neglect them. *Alternating Currents.*—Still another class of currents is to be considered. In the induction coil, and in certain types of dynamo machines, the variations of the current are very much more marked than in any case we have so far looked into.

The details of the apparatus giving such currents will be more fully described further on. At present we may simply say that the machine itself actuates two circuits,—the "primary " and the "secondary,"—so arranged relatively to each other that any variation or change in the "primary" circuit produces a corresponding change in the " secondary. " In general, the primary current is reversed, *i.e.*, driven first in one direction, then in the opposite, a definite number of times per minute, and the secondary current follows the same order of change.

In a particular case the current will be represented by the curve given in Fig. 28, though often it is not nearly so regular as here shown. However, what it is desired to make clear is that the current fluctuates between fixed values on both sides of the zero line; that is to say, after the current has reached its greatest value at A it falls to zero at B, after which it reaches again a maximum value at C, but in the opposite direction to its former one. Thus, the current continually changes from a given intensity in one direction to the same intensity in the opposite direction, and at a certain instant between these two epochs it becomes really zero. Currents furnished by an ordinary RhumkorfF coil are of this nature, and, indeed, the same is true of nearly all forms of induction apparatus.

The word "current" is always used in the sense of Current Strength or Current Intensity, but it is best to define it as the *quantity* of electricity passing through a section of the conductor in the unit time; that is, if there are Q units of electricity going through any cross-section of the circuit in a time represented by t seconds, then

Current = —

We can say any section, because the current in one part of a continuous circuit is equal to the current in any other part. The electric current obeys the law of continuity, according to which the total quantity of electricity in the universe cannot be increased or diminished. Thus, if we have a circuit made up as in Fig. 29, in which A is a coiled iron wire, B a stout bar of copper, G an ordinary galvanometer, C a coiled piece of copper wire, F a silver voltameter, and Dx and $D2$ cells furnishing the current, then we shall always find that the galvanometer and voltameter register the same current.

Xo matter in what portion of the circuit we place the galvanometer, and wherever we insert the voltameter, provided hoth are directly in the path of the current, the latter, as measured by the two instruments will always be the same. Indeed, it is in consequence of this fact that we are enabled to standardize current measuring instruments by the use of the voltameter.

Ohm's Law.—Suppose we have an arrangement of any kind that will furnish us with a steady current, and let the current flow through a certain length of ordinary copper wire. Let us include in the circuit some instrument—a *galvanometer*— which will measure the current passing through it. Suppose, further, that we have another instrument, such as an *electrometer*, which will measure differences of potential or electromotive forces; and let us attach to the two electrodes of this a pair of wires, which can be

Fig. 29.

brought in contact with the circuit conductor at different points along its length. AVe will assume that the conductor referred to, and shown in Fig. 30 as $A E$, is of uniform section. The arrangement will be something like that given in the figure. Let the wire be divided into any convenient number of equal parts, and for the first experiment let us place the ends $Pl\ P0$ (connected with the electrometer V) in contact with the points A and B. Suppose the galvanometer indicates a value K for the current, and let the electrometer show a difference of potential or electro-motive force equal to i?1 so that Vx is the potential at A and $V2$ the potential at B; then $Ex = Vx-Va$.

Suppose, now, that the current remaining constant, we keep Pi still in contact with A, but move P2 along the wire until it reaches C. $A B$ and $B C$ being equal lengths, we shall observe that the electrometer gives a value for the difference of potential twice as great as before, namely, $E2 = 2\ Ex$. Again, at D it will be three times as great and at E four times as great, and so on indefinitely, according to the number of sections.

Now, keeping everything as it was before, let us simply double the source of electricity; that is, if we had one cell in use before, let us replace it by two similar cells,—preferably storage cells, for a reason to be explained later. The current, as shown by the galvanometer, will be twice as great as at first, and the difference of potential between the points A and E will also be doubled. We observe, then, that the current, other things being equal, is doubled when the electro-motive force is doubled; in other words, it is directly proportional to the electro-motive force.

Now replace the wire $A E$ by a similar wire twice as long. and observe again the current. It will be found to have fallen to its original value, notwithstanding the fact that the electromotive force is higher. If, instead of having doubled the length of wire we had allowed this to remain the same, but had halved its cross-sectional area, we should have obtained the same result. It appears, therefore, that the wire opposes the flow of the current, and the more effectually the greater its length and the smaller its diameter. It is. in consequence, said to offer " resistance "to the passage of electricity, and, from the experiment given above, it appears that the current is smaller, the electromotive force remaining the same, the greater the resistance of the wire through which it flows.

We could continue the experiment and prove the same thing for all sizes and lengths of wire and for different values of the electro-motive force, but enough has been done to establish a relation between the quantities, current, electromotive force, and resistance. This relation is expressed by the statement that *the current in any conductor is equal to (lie electromotive force between its ends divided by its resistance;* or, symbolically,

«-!

and the law itself is known as Ohm's Law.

In the above experiment we have assumed that the resistance of the battery itself could be neglected, since we assumed that simply doubling the electromotive force would double the current; but this is not always true. In general, the resistance of the battery being considerable,—unless we use a storage cell,—it cannot be ignored; and in practice we shall find that the current is less than it would be under the hypothesis. Thus, in the particular case given above, if we suppose the electrometer disconnected, to apply Ohm's law we should have to write $C = Rx + Ra + R3 + R$ where E is the electro-motive force of the battery, Rx its own (internal) resistance, $ll2$ the resistance of the galvanometer, $R\$$ of the divided wire, and i?4 of all the connections taken together. Hence it is only when the total sum $R + R2 + \text{-}\#i$ is very small in comparison with $R3$ that we double the current in $A E$ by doubling the electro-motive force of the source.

The experiments we have just supposed made show us that the resistance opposed by any body—in this case a metal wire —to the now of electricity through it depends upon the length of the conductor, increasing as this increases, and, upon the sectional area, diminishing as this increases. That is to say, for a given metal the resistance is proportional to the length of the wire and inversely proportional to the area; we can write, therefore, $I\ I\ R = K$-or $= K\ a\ 7i,.2\ /$ being the length of the wire, a its sectional area, and r its radius, so that $a = n\ r2$. K is a constant, depending upon the nature of the conductor. If we should continue these experiments and should observe the effects of using wires of different metals, we should find that the resistance depends not only upon the length and sectional area of the conductor, but also upon the nature of the material as well. Thus, the resistance of an iron wire is about six times as great as that of a similar copper conductor; this means that with the same electro-motive force a current six times as great will flow through a copper bar as through an iron bar in all respects identical.

It has become necessary, therefore, to adopt some metal as a standard and to compare other conductors with it, just as in the determination of specific gravities the density of every substance is referred to that of water, whose density is assumed to be unity. The same thing has been done in this case, and silver in a chemically pure state has been selected as a standard of reference, which forms a basis for the comparison of the resistance of other metals.

The resistance of a given substance is affected by still another circumstance besides its length, sectional area, and its metallic peculiarity, namely, it depends upon the temperature. In all cases, so far as known, the resistance of conductors increases as the temperature rises. The resistance of so-called non-conductors, such as gutta-percha, glass, etc., however, diminishes with increase of temperature, and the same thing is true for all electrolytes.

The relation between the resistance and the temperature of metals has been very carefully investigated, and it has been found that between the limits of 0 and 100 C. the increase of resistance with increase of temperature is very regular for any one metal, but that it varies considerably for different metals. If we call q the increase in the unit resistance for 1 C. rise in temperature, $R0$ the resistance of the wire at 0 C, and fit its resistance at a temperature (t), then i?, $= R0\ (1 + q\ t)$.

Hence, to make the foregoing formula perfectly general we must write $Bt = (1 + q\ 0 ——S.\ 71\ ra\ Ii,,$ being the resistance of unit length and unit cross-section. This is generally called the specific resistance.

In some respects the electric current may be compared to the flow of water through a channel; that is, the current of electricity obeys the laws of an incompressible fluid, and hence the *quantity of electricity* for each unit area may be greater at some parts of a given section of the. channel than at others. Since we understand by the quantity of electricity flowing through the unit area the density of the current, we may say that the current density is variable at different points in the circuit. Wherever and from whatever cause the path of the current is confined within narrow limits, there the density of the current will be greatest, and *vice versa.* When the current density is great its path is necessarily restricted, and hence the resistance of the circuit is greater than it would be for a smaller density.

Advantage of this fact is sometimes taken in the application of electricity to the human body, by varying the size of the electrodes through which the current passes. When it is desired to make the resistance offered to the current very small the practice is to use electrodes—moistened pieces of sponge, etc., fastened to metal plates—of large surface, and small electrodes for larger resistances. In this way the area through which the current passes can be varied, and, therefore, with it the density of the current.

KirchhofFs Laws.—From what has been said previously it appears that the resistance of any circuit is equal to the sum of the resistances of its parts. If, for instance, we join end to end two similar wires of the same metal, the resistance of this part of the circuit will be twice as great as before. Suppose, however, that we place the wires side by side, as in Fig. 31. The result in this case—assuming that the wires are exactly similar—will be that the resistance between the points A B will become half of what it was with a single wire. The current has now two paths in which to travel, and since the paths are alike it will be "resisted" only half as strongly as if there were but a single path. There is a good analogy to this in the case of water flowing from a tank or reservoir through pipes. If the tank has only one outlet the flow of water will be half as great as if it had two identical openings, and so on for any number. We assume, of course, that the outlets are all on the same level, so that the pressure is the same at the different openings.

Extending the principle, we see that the resistance between any two points will diminish in the ratio of the number of conductors joining the points. If, therefore, we have any number of wires (Fig. 32), with resistances, $Ru\ R\%$ up to Rn joining any two points A and $B)$ whose difference of potential is $E,$ we have, in all cases,

Where $Cl,\ C2...\ Cn$ are the currents in the wires, $Rly\ R2$ Rn respectively. Adding these, we have

If we write for the sum

The quantity $/$ is called the resultant

resistance of the circuit, and is ' equal to the sum of the reciprocals of the different resistances of which the circuit between the points is composed. Since, however, the reciprocal of resistance is conductivity, we may say that the resultant conductivity of a circuit between two given points is equal to the sum of the separate conductivities of the wires joining these points.

'Wires joined in this way, *i.e.*, side by side, are said to be connected in "parallel" or in multiple arc. In the case of two wires we have $r\ Rx\ T\ R3$ or, $1\ Rx + Ra$ or, what amounts to the same thing, $i + Ra$ that is, *the resultant resistance is equal to the product of the two separate resistances divided by their sum.*

Hence, if the wires are equal, $Rx = R\%$ and $2\ Rx\ 2$ *i.e.*, the resistance is half as great as before. For three wires $r\ Rx\ Ra\ R3$ or the resistance has become one-third as great as it was for a single wire. In the general case of n wires we have
_ $R1\ R3\ R3\ Rn\ Rx\ Ra... Rw.1\ \text{-f}\ Rr\ R3...$
$RH\text{--}R3\ Ra... RK$

This may be expressed by saying that the resultant resistance of any number (») of conductors joined in parallel is equal to the product of all the n resistances, divided by the sum of all the products which can be formed by multiplying $n — i$ of the resistances together. This is known,as the law of multiple conductors.

The foregoing statement regarding the continuity of electric currents may be put into another form. We may express the same thing by saying that the algebraic sum of all the currents at a point is zero; that is, if we call the currents flowing *toward a* point (Fig. 33) positive, and those going *away* from it negative, then the sum of all the positive currents is equal to the sum of all the negative currents, and hence, if we add these, the result is zero. This is known as *KirclJioJf's first law,* and is generally written symbolically thus:— where the sign 2 means simply summation, due regard being given to the signs.

Let us now consider a circuit in which there are several sources of electro-motive force (Fig. 34). Let the resistances of the various sources be so small that we may neglect them, and call the resistances of the connecting wires $Ru\ 7?2i\ i?3i\ B$ as shown; further designate the potential at various points along the circuit by $PA, PB,$ etc. We can then apply Ohm's law to the case in the following way: If we call the currents in the different wires $Cu\ C$ etc., we have $C1R1 = PA\text{-}PB, Csr = Pc—pd, G3R3 = PE—Pf,.$
$CE, = P6\text{-}P,,$

Adding these, we obtain $Cx\ Rl + C2\ Ra + C3\ Ba + CtRt = (PA\text{-}PB) + (Pc\text{-}PD) + (PB\text{-}PF)+ (Pe\text{-}PB)$

The quantities on thewight-hand side $(PA — PB$ etc.) are the differences of potential in the sources of electro-motive forces themselves, and for these we can therefore write, respectively, $EK\ E\ E\ E\pm$ The equation then becomes $El + E3 + E3 + Et = (7,\ i?,\ + C3\ R3 + C3\ R3 + Ct\ Rt$ which can also be written $2£ = 2\ C\ R;$ that is, the sum of all the electro-motive forces in any circuit is equal to the sum of all the products obtained by multiplying the separate currents by the resistances through which they are flowing. This is known as *Kirclthoff second law.*

Where we have a complete circuit, as in the figure, it is evident that, instead of $C\ C\%$ etc., we can use a single term G to express the sum of the values of the currents, since the same current must flow through all parts as a whole. The preceding thus becomes $2\ E = C\ 2\ R$

KirchhofFs laws are of great value in the consideration of many electrical problems in which complex and divided circuits are involved. Let us take, for instance, the case of *Whealstone's bridge. Wheatstone's Bridge.*—Suppose we have six conductors, joined up as in Fig. 35. Let there be inserted between the points B and C a galvanometer, and between the points A and D a battery, the resistance of the two, with connections, etc., being designated respectively by K and R. Suppose that the current flows in the direction from D to A through the battery, and let the potential at B be greater than that at $C,$ *i.e.,* call the difference of potential between B and A (that is, $B — A)$ positive, so that the-current flows as shown in the figure. Then

Fig. 35. Fig. 38.
we have, by KirchhofFs first law, calling G the current through the galvanometer, and //that through the battery, $\# = Ca\text{-}(.\ C4i\ G = (\ — Cti\ G = C — C3$

From the second law, we obtain in the circuits $ABC, BCD,$ etc.,

It follows, therefore, that if we know the value, in any system of units, of one of the resistances, $Ru\ R\ R$ or $R4$ and the *ratio* of any two of the remaining three, we can determine the value of the other at once in the same system of units. Thus, suppose we know that $RA = 10$ units, and suppose, further, we find by actual experiment that $7?t: R2 = 5;$ then we have $\text{-"}a$ as the preceding equation may be written, and, substituting the values just given, we get $R = 10 \times 5 = 50$ units.

In its usual form, Wheatstone's bridge consists of a wire of uniform section, $C\ D$ (Fig. 36), stretched alongside a scale, divided generally into a hundred equal parts. This wire is connected with the resistances to be measured by means of a pair of heavy copper bars, $H\ H$ provided with binding posts, to which the coils $R3$ and RA may be fastened. These bars are made of large section, so that their resistance may be very small compared with that to be measured. The third bar, $H3$ is used to connect the resistances under experiment together, and to make a contact for the galvanometer.

$R3$ and RA represent the known and unknown resistances, respectively. B is the battery, joined up as shown, and G is the galvanometer. One contact of the latter is *fixed* between the resistances $R3$ and $i?,$ and one is variable, the point P being movable along the wire $C\ D$ until the two parts into which it is thus divided establish the sought-for equilibrium. This happens when the two lengths of the wire $C\ D$ arc in the same ratio as the resistances on corresponding sides, $R3$ and $i?4$ and under these circumstances *there will be no current through the galvanometer.* Suppose, for instance, that $R3$ is 35 units, and that the point P occupies such a position as to divide the wire $C\ D$ into two parts, whose lengths are

1G and 84, the former length being on the left-hand side; then we have at once 16:84 = 35: *x;* whence, 84 X 35 10 183. 75 units.

The wire *C D* must be of uniform section in order that we may assume the resistances of its two parts to be proportional to their lengths, which would not be true if the wire were thicker at one point than at another.

Heating Effects of the Current.—We have shown (page 30) that the energy of a charge of electricity is proportional to the *quantity* of electricity in the charge multiplied by its *potential.* In a similar way we can prove that the energy of a current of electricity is proportional to the product of the *quantity* of electricity flowing multiplied by the *electro-motive force* under which it flows; that is, if we have a current, *C,* in a circuit whose electro-motive force is *E* flowing during a time, *t,* the energy given out in this time is *Cut* or we may say that the Rate at which Energy is "*given out* is *C E.* If the conditions outside the circuit remain the same (the circuit itself being unchanged) this energy is all converted into heat; and if, therefore, the product *C E t* represents *energy,* we must multiply this by a factor to determine the *heat generated.* This factor is called the dynamical equivalent of heat, and represents the number of units of heat which are equivalent to the unit of work or energy. The former is that quantity of heat which will raise the temperature of one pound of water one degree centigrade, and the latter, written J", has been carefully determined by Joule and others.

From Ohm's law we can write the product *C E* in either of two ways. Since *E* we have, by substituting for *G* in the equation just given, the expression

That is, the heat generated is equal to the square of the electromotive force multiplied by the time the current was flowing, divided by the resistance, and divided by Joule's equivalent, *J.* Or, since *E = C R,* we obtain, by substituting *C R* for *E, H= C Rt* 4 which can be stated thus: The heat generated by the current, *C,* flowing during the time, *t,* is equal to the square of the *current* multiplied by the *resistance,* multiplied by the *time,* and *divided* by J, as before. Any one of these formulae may be used indiscriminately, and in a particular case we employ that form which contains only such of the quantities *C, R,* and *E* as are given or known.

Thus, if we know both the current and the electro-motive force, we use the first equation. If we do not know the value of the current, but have the electro-motive force and resistance given, we employ the second formula, and so on.

These laws apply to a part of a complete circuit as well as to the entire circuit. Thus, if we know the resistance, *R,* in any part of a circuit (Fig. 37) in which a current, *C,* is flowing,

'then we have, for the rate at which heat is generated *in that particular part* of the circuit, Ca R

If, in another part, we do not know the resistance (i?2), but' find the potential at the ends of this part to be *Vx* and *l* we have for the rate of generation of heat, as before, (*V%*-Fa) *C*

These formulae will be found very useful in their application to the actual cautery and to the calculation of the heating effects in the various surgical devices which are raised to a high temperature by means of the electric current.

Electrolysis.—When a current is made to flow through a liquid a chemical change will in most cases be found to occur at the points where the current enters and where it leaves the liquid. This change will be different in different cases; it may consist in the liberation of a gas at one or both of these points, or in the deposition or solution of a metal. Thus, if we dip two platinum plates (Fig. 38) in a vessel of ordinary undistilled water and attach the plates by means of a wire with the poles of a sufficiently strong battery, we shall notice in a short time that gas bubbles are beginning to form on both of the plates. If the current is much increased the gas bubbles will be formed in such quantities that they will become detached from the surface of the plates and will rise to the top of the liquid.

If, instead of using ordinary water, we had immersed the plates in a solution of sulphate of copper, we should have found that the plate through which the current *left* the liquid was covered with a deposit of copper, which, under favorable circumstances, would be in the form of a bright metallic film, while the other plate remained unchanged. In this case, with a current not too strong, we should have observed no evolution of gas at either plate; but if by a careful analysis or other means we had accurately determined the amount of copper present as sulphate in the solution, we should have found it diminished by the exact amount deposited on the platinum plate after the passage of the current. Further than this, if we had used a *copper* plate instead of the *platinum* plate *which we found unaffected* we should have observed this to lose in weight exactly-what the platinum plate gained; but in this case the strength of copper-sulphate solution would remain unchanged.

This action of the electric current is universal, and we always find that the solution through which the current passes tends to become weaker while one plate gains a definite amount of metal, the gain on one side and the loss on the other being exactly equivalent. It is always found that the metal is deposited in a certain way relatively to the direction of the current; that is, only the plate through which the current leaves the solution receives a deposit; and, furthermore, it is found that the weight of metal so deposited is exactly proportional to the whole quantity of electricity which has passed through the solution. These phenomena, included under the term ElecTrolysis, have been subjected to very careful study and measurement, and their laws have been quite fully investigated.

Faraday called the positive plate—*i. e.,* the plate through which the current enters the liquid—the *anode,* the negative plate the *kathode,* both together being called indefinitely *electrodes.* The solution through which the current flows is called an *electrolyte,* the substance deposited on the negative plate—generally a metal—being the *Jeathion,* that deposited on the positive plate the *anion,* and both products of decomposition being *ions*. These terms are now very generally used.

Polarization.—In the experiment cited above, of passing a current through two platinum plates dipping in water, we shall observe that the strength of the current rapidly diminishes after a few minutes, and unless the galvanometer we are using is extremely sensitive the current in a short time will apparently cease altogether. If we now break the circuit and take out the battery, then join the two plates by a wire, including a galvanometer, we shall observe a current in the *opposite* direction to the former, which also, after a very short time, will become too small to be perceptible. This diminution of the primary current and production of a reverse current is due to a single cause,— the action of the gas condensed on the surface of the electrodes. The action has led some experimenters to affirm that Ohm's law does not hold in this case. Such statements seem, however, to be unwarranted, and later investigation has shown that Ohm's law is just as true for electrolytic conduction as for any other. In other words, it appears that the gas on the electrodes sets up a reverse electromotive force, which, acting in the opposite direction to that of the decomposing current, diminishes the effect of this until finally the current itself becomes so small as to be unnoticeable. Moreover, the phenomenon is Aery seriously affected by the quality of the water used, and it is found that with very pure water in the electrolytic cell a very much greater electro-motive force is required than if we had used ordinary undistilled water.

The phenomena just mentioned are not evident when absolutely pure water containing dilute sulphuric acid and perfectly clean platinum plates are used in connection with a small electromotive force. In this case it is found that after a very short time the current actuallv vanishes. Disturbing effects are due to the presence of free hydrogen and oxygen gas in the liquid itself; but if under the conditions referred to,—*i.e.,* if we employ chemically-pure substances,— then no discrepancies arise.

The gases present on the plates (and a certain amount can always be found) seem to be much more intimately associated with the metal than would result from mere condensation, and seem to show something of the nature of a chemical combination.

In all cases of electrolysis it is found that the weight of substance decomposed by a given current is always the same for that substance, whatever may be the chemical state in which it occurs. Thus, if we allow the unit current to flow for one minute through a solution of silver nitrate the amount of silver deposited on the anode will be the same as if we had employed fused, silver chloride or any other salt of silver in such a state as to allow the passage of the electric current. It has also been observed that the quantity of substance decomposed by the unit current in the unit time—that is, one second—bears.a pertain definite relation to the atomic weight of the substance, and the quantity of an element set free under these circumstances—that is, by the unit current in one second—is called the electrochemical equivalent of the substance.

From this it follows that if we know the atomic weight of any element and the electro-chemical equivalent of some other substance which may be taken as a standard of reference, we can calculate either the quantity of electricity which has flowed through the substance (supposed in solution and its weight known), or we can determine the weight decomposed by the current when we know the value of the current and the length of time it has been flowing. On this fact depends the accuracy and usefulness of an instrument called the *voltameter,* which is extensively employed as a means of standardizing current measuring instruments.

It has been stated that electrolytic conduction takes place in accordance with Ohm's law as truly as does ordinary metallic conduction. Yet apparent discrepancies exist, and the explanation is difficult, even impossible, unless all attending circumstances are taken into consideration. An apparent difficulty is the action before referred to, which reduces the current flowing through an electrolyte after it has been running a short time, until it finally ceases altogether. It has been found as stated, however, that the reduction in the intensity of the current is due to an opposing or Counter *electromotive force,* so that we have acting in the circuit not the electromotive force of the source itself, but the difference between this and the counter electromotive force set up in the voltameter. If we should carefully determine this difference, and then measure the current, we should find that Ohm's law is rigorously true in this case, as in all others.-Thus, if E is the electromotive force of the source, e that of the voltameter (negative because in the opposite direction to E), we have A voltameter (Fig. 38) is simply a yessel containing a very pure solution of some metallic salt (nitrate of silver or sulphate of copper being most frequently used), in which dip two plates of pure metal. Sometimes a metallic vessel is employed, this constituting itself one electrode. By weighing one electrode before and after the passage of the current, thus determining the loss or gain in weight, for a given number of minutes, the current which has flowed can be calculated at once.

$$\text{Current} = \frac{E-e}{r}$$

r being the total resistance.

In order to explain the phenomenon of electrolysis several hypotheses have been advanced, the most noteworthy of which is, perhaps, the theory of Clausius, which can be given in the following way:—

"According to the theory of molecular motion, of which Clausius himself has been the chief founder, every molecule of the fluid is moving in an exceedingly irregular manner, being driven first one way and then the other by the impact of molecules, which are also in a state of agitation.

"This molecular agitation goes on at all times independently of the action of electro-motive force. The diffusion of one fluid through another is brought about by this molecular agitation, which increases in velocity as the temperature rises. The agitation being exceedingly irregular, the encounters of the molecules take place with various degrees of violence, and it is probable that even at low temperatures some of the encounters are so violent that one or both of the component molecules are split up into their constituents. Each of these constituent molecules then knocks about among the rest until it meets with another molecule of the opposite kind, with which it unites to form a new molecule of the compound. In every compound, therefore, a certain proportion of the molecules at any instant are broken up into their constituent atoms. At high temperatures the proportion becomes so large as to produce the phenomenon of dissociation.

"Now, Clausius supposes that it is on the constituent molecules in their intervals of freedom that the electro-motive force acts, deflecting them slightly from the paths which they would otherwise have followed, and causing the positive constituents to travel, on the whole, more in the positive than in the negative direction, and the negative constituents more in the negative than in the positive direction. The electro-motive force does not, therefore, produce the disruptions and reunions of the molecules, but, rinding these disruptions and reunions already going on, it influences the motion of the constituents during their intervals of freedom. The amount of this influence is proportional to the electro-motive force when the temperature is given. The higher the temperature, however, the greater the molecular agitation and the more numerous are the free constituents." Hence, the electro-motive force has more atoms on which to act, and there is a more rapid evolution of gas at the surfaces of the electrodes. This also explains why the conductivity of electrolytes increases with increase of temperature.

Clausius' explanation of electrolysis seems to accord with what is known experimentally better than any other which has yet been put forward, and the theory of molecular agitation on which it depends is the foundation of the so-called kinetic theory of gases now very generally accepted.

Maxwell, "Elec. and Mag."

CHAPTER II.

Magnetism.

Magnetism was first discovered by the ancients as a property of a now well-known and widely-scattered mineral called the *loadstone,* which is an oxide of iron of the composition Fe_3O_4.

It has long been known that if we dip a fragment of load stone into a mass of iron filings the filings will cling to the latter, and that they will adhere in greater numbers at certain particular regions than at others. These regions are sometimes well defined, and we shall observe that there are always two spots, usually the ends, whose properties are of an opposite character (as in the case of bodies charged with electricity), separated by an interval of little or even no action at all.

That the opposite ends of a piece of natural magnet, as we may call the loadstone, possess really opposite properties can be shown in many ways. If we allow the needle of an ordinary compass (Fig. 39) to come to rest and approach one end of the loadstone to it, it will move, and, let us suppose, it is repelled. After it has again come to rest turn the loadstone end for end and bring it near the needle again; the needle will be attracted. If we take a rod of rather hard iron and rub one end over one extremity of the loadstone and the other end over the other extremity, we shall observe a similar phenomenon in the iron so treated. Again, let us rub one end of a bar of iron with end *A* of the loadstone (Fig. 40), one end over *B.* Treat another bar in a similar way. Then we shall find that the ends, both of which have been rubbed with *A* or *B,* repel each otlier, and that the ends rubbed with *A* attract the ends rubbed with *B; i.e.,* like ends repel, unlike attract, exactly as we have already found in the case of electricity.

The ends of a piece of loadstone, or of a bar of iron or steel, rubbed by it are called the *magnetic poles,* and the opposite extremities are distinguished by the names *north* and *south* poles. This, as in electricity, in which we distinguish between positive and negative, is merely a matter of convention.

It is well known that if we suspend a piece of loadstone so that it is free to turn it will take up a definite position relatively to certain fixed directions on the earth's surface; and that a rod of steel or hard iron which has been acted upon by a natural magnet, which we may, therefore, call an artificial magnet, will act in a similar manner. One end of the magnet will turn in a northerly direction, though not exactly north, and this end is by common acceptation called the north pole, the south pole, of course, being at the opposite end.

The *mariner's compass,* without which modern navigation would be an impossibility, is simply an artificial magnet suspended on a pivot and free to turn, with very little friction, in a horizontal plane.

As in electricity, so in magnetism, it is necessary to speak of quantity, and the unit quantity of magnetism, or unit pole, is simply a matter of definition to which other quantities are referred.

The unit pole is defined as that pole which will repel another similar pole, placed at the unit distance from it, with a unit force. Thus, its value depends upon the system of fundamental units; namely, of length, of time, and of mass which we may have adopted.

If, in accordance with the notation of electrical quantities, we call north magnetism plus (+) and south magnetism minus (—), then, also, we may show that the total quantity of magnetism in any magnet, with due regard to signs, is zero. The idea of two magnetic fluids is also useful in some cases, but we must remember that it is only for convenience that it is adopted, and to more readily explain the action of magnets and magnetic bodies. Thus, it is often assumed that there is a distribution of these magnetic fluids over the surface of every magnet, and that the quantity present on the surface varies from place to place. It is, therefore, very similar to the distribution of electricity over the surface of conductors. If by any appropriate means we determine this magnetic distribution, for instance, very roughly, by dipping a bar magnet in iron filings, and observing where the filings are most dense, we shall find it to resemble that shown in Fig. 41. Thus, the filings will adhere very much more strongly at the ends, and their density will gradually diminish as we approach the central region, until, when we reach the centre itself, there is no effect observable at all. We assume, then, that the magnetic fluids present on the magnet—plus at one end, minus at the other—are concentrated at the ends, and that the centre is a neutral region, as shown in the figure, where the curves represent the apparent density of magnetic fluid along the length of the magnet.

Total Quantity of Magnetism is Zero.— If we break a magnet of any form whatever it might be thought from the preceding that, if the fracture should occur at the middle part, there will be no magnetism at these ends. Such, however, is not the case; and the magnetism at the broken surfaces will be the same in quantity as at the original ends,—similarly in every respect to what we have found to occur in electric distribution. If the magnet in Fig. 42 is broken in halves, each piece will form a magnet as strong, or nearly as strong, as the original magnet. And generally, if a magnet is broken up into any number of pieces, each of them will form a magnet of the same strength as the original magnet itself. When joined together again by their fractured surfaces, the original magnet will be reproduced. For, suppose the magnet XS is broken up into four pieces, as shown in Fig. 42, we may consider that at any point of the original magnet there are equal quantities of X and S magnetism present, and that, being equal and opposite, their total effect is zero. This is really the case when the broken magnet is restored by joining the fragments together. For at every fractured surface there are equal X and S poles, which neutralize each other; and hence the only effective magnetism is that at the ends, which is practically the same in quantity now as before the magnet was ruptured.

It might seem that this was contrary to the law of the conservation of energy, inasmuch as it might appear that energy is created by the process. A little reflection, however, shows us that this is only apparently true, since the fragments of the broken magnet are not themselves magnets until they are separated, and in the act of separating them we do an amount of work equal to that which they could do by attracting other magnets.

Lines of Magnetic Force.— In the explanation of electrical attractions and repulsions we made use of Faraday's idea of lines of force. In the study of magnetism we shall find the conception of very much greater value, and shall at once realize how materially it will aid us in the understanding of many magnetic and electro-magnetic phenomena of the utmost importance.

According to Faraday's view every magnet is supposed to send outward from itself " lines of force" into the surrounding region. Starting from one pole, they go outward a certain distance, and then, curving backward in a more or less regular manner, they finally reach the opposite pole. The general directions of these lines of force for an ordinary bar magnet are exhibited with sufficient accuracy in Fig. 43. Fig. 44 shows the lines of force around the poles of a horse-shoe magnet. They can be easily obtained by dropping iron filings on a piece of card-board held over the poles of the magnet. Under these circumstances the little particles of iron become themselves magnets, and direct themselves according to the direction of the magnetic force at the points they occupy. By slightly tapping the card the particles are shifted about and are enabled to group themselves more readily, which they do in a very regular manner. The lines of force are, therefore, the directions which a magnet would take up, if freely suspended so that it could rotate under the action of the existing magnetic

Fig. 43.
Fig. 44.

force. The region itself in which these lines of force exist, *i.e.,* the space surrounding a magnet, is called the *magnetic field,* and if we know at every point the direction and number of the lines of force the field is completely defined. For we may take the number of lines of force within any given area as a measure of the relative intensity of the magnetic force within that area.

These two ways of regarding the phenomenon of magnetic distribution are really alike, for the density of the so-called magnetic fluids over a magnet corresponds with the relative number of lines of force issuing from its surface at different points. Thus, at the poles, where we have supposed the magnetic fluids to accumulate, there the lines of force issuing are greatest in number, and this can be shown experimentally. Near the centre there are no lines of force, which is in agreement with the hypothesis that here the magnetic fluid is also absent.

Indeed, we could determine the magnetic distribution from the number of lines of force by supposing a unit of magnetism to give rise to a certain number of lines of force, which we could take as the unit for comparison.

The law which determines the intensity of the attraction and repulsion between two magnets is not so easy to prove as the corresponding law in electricity; for we cannot separate one pole of a magnet from the other, that is, we cannot separate the two kinds of magnetism from each other. We can, however, approximate to this by using long, thin magnets; for then, the poles being nearly at the ends, are far enough apart to be studied separately. In a manner similar to the method of experiment adopted by Coulomb it is found that the attraction between two dissimilar poles is equal to the product of the strength of the poles (that is, the product of the quantities of magnetism) divided by the distance between them, squared, exactly as in the case of electricity.

Earth a Large Magnet— As is well known, a magnet, when freely suspended, away from other magnets, will assume always a definite direction, relatively to the geographical meridian at the place. This is due to the action of the earth, wdiich has in consequence been compared to a large magnet, and the directions of its lines of force over the greater part of the globe have been carefully studied and mapped out. *Horizontal and Vertical Components of the Earth's Force.—* There are always to be considered two components of the earth's magnetic force—a horizontal and a vertical component, both of which exert an action on a freely-suspended magnet. The horizontal component is, however, much more important in electrical work than the vertical, since it is this foree only which can affect most electrical measuring instruments. This is on account of the way in which the magnetic needle is suspended, which does not permit any movement in a vertical plane.

The direction of the earth's horizontal force is not always the same relatively to the meridian lines on its surface; that is, the magnet does not point due north and south, and it also varies in the same place from time to time. This deviation from a true north and south orientation, at any point, is called the magnetic declination at that point, and occasionally the declination is very marked, amounting to many degrees in some cases. The general direction of the lines of force themselves at any locality is called the "magnetic meridian."

The action of the earth on a suspended magnet is simply a tendency to cause rotation—if the magnet is displaced from its normal position—and there is no tendency whatever to cause a movement of the magnet as a whole, because the effect on the two poles are exactly equal and opposite. If the magnet is deflected from its normal position— that is, from the magnetic meridian—the force with which it is pulled back varies as the sine of the angle of rotation, not with the angle itself. It is greater the longer the magnet, and the stronger its magnetic poles.

A magnetic field in which the lines of force are parallel and at equal distances apart is called a uniform field (Fig. *4x*). Such a field—at least throughout the small space which we ever have occasion to consider at any one time—is thatof the earth, but it is seldom that we can produce a field of this sort artificially, and then only throughout a very limited area.

*Magnetic Induction.—*We have heretofore considered only such magnetic bodies as the loadstone itself or bodies which have been rendered magnetic by being rubbed with a piece of loadstone. A bar of steel, or rather hard iron, magnetized in this way, is said to be *magnetized hy induction,* and the phenomenon is of very mucb the same kind as that of electrification by induction. But in the latter case the electrification completely disappears on the removal of the inducing body, while here the magnetism is always more or less permanent. If we bring a piece of hard iron near a natural magnet (Fig. 46) the direction of the lines of force due to the latter is changed in such a way as to make a certain number pass through the iron itself (Fig. 47). The iron is said to be a better conductor for the lines of magnetic force than the air, and the lines therefore tend to pass, through the iron as much as possible. This is shown in the figures. In the first we have the normal distribution of mag Except along two line drawn on tut earth's surface, which are called lines of no deviation. netism shown by the direction of the lines of force issuing from the poles JVand *S.* In the latter we observe how these directions have become changed, and how a number of lines, instead of passing directly backward from the north pole to the south pole, enter first the iron rod, proceed a certain distance through this, and then, issuing from its end and sides, curve backward and terminate at the south pole of the loadstone. uWe also observe, assuming that the lines of force have their origin at the north pole of the loadstone, that where they enter the iron rod a south pole is developed, the north pole being indefinitely located near the farther extremity.

If the loadstone is now removed the magnetism that remains re-adjusts itself, and the lines of force assume their normal form, the poles being at or near the ends. The intensity of the magnetization after the removal of the loadstone is not the same under all circumstances, but depends upon the nature of the magnetized body. AVe have supposed steel or hard iron used in the experiments just mentioned, and under these circumstances v,he magnetic effect is quite permanent. It is not absolutely constant; indeed, it diminishes considerably at the instant the magnetizing force is removed, but after that it changes under favorable conditions very little. If we had used a soil-iron rod, however, scarcely any residual magnetism would have been observable after the loadstone had been removed to a distance. Soft iron is very much easier to magnetize than hard iron or steel, and is also very much easier to demagnetize, and this property is closely related to the *physical hardness* or *softness* of the material. According to Weber's theory of magnetism, the *particles* of iron and steel are supposed to rotate under the action of the magnetic force, so that their poles assume all the same direction. In a bar of iron not subject to magnetic force the particles are situated indefinitely as regards direction,—on the whole, as many pointing one way as the opposite. Magnetic force tends to turn these all in the same direction, so that the effects are added together, and in hard iron and steel the molecules, once rotated, do not easily regain their former directions, but remain as they are. However, the intensity of this residual magnetism, as it is called, is really a matter of degree. The hardest steel gradually loses some of its magnetism (it may be very little), and the softest iron always retains some traces of the magnetic forces which have acted upon it. There are other bodies besides iron and steel which are susceptible of magnetic influence in a marked degree. Such are nickel and cobalt, but their magnetic power is very small compared with that of iron and steel. It is not possible to magnetize very strongly a rod of iron by means of the loadstone. Very much more powerful effects can be secured by the action of an electric current, which, indeed, is universally employed in practice for this purpose.

Magnetic Action of the Electric Current. —In 1841 Oersted discovered that a magnet suspended near a wire in which was flowing a current of electricity was

acted upon by the current in such a way as to cause it to assume a certain definite position relatively to the current. lie found that if the current was passed along a straight wire (Fig. 48), and the magnet was near this, the latter tended to place itself at right angles to the current, the north pole always pointing in one way relatively to the direction of the current. The rule for finding the direction in which the north pole will move is as follows: If the current flows from S to X, and is over the magnet, the north pole will move always to the west. On further investigation Oersted found that the angle through which the needle turned, L supposing it originally in the s
Fig. 48. Fig. 49.
magnetic meridian, was dependent upon the strength of the current, and upon the proximity of this to the magnet. The stronger the current, and the smaller the distance between this and the magnet, the greater the angular deflection.

To understand this action-of an electric current, which may be called a magnetic action, we must again attempt to form a mental picture of the state of things in the medium surroundinsr the wire. We have alreadv seen how the lines of force exist around electrified bodies and around magnets, and with some slight modifications exactly the same thing is true for electric currents, or rather for the region about the current.

But the lines of force around a long, straight wire carrying a current are circular (Fig. 49); they are continuous, and cannot be said to end nor to begin at any point. That is to say, at any point near a straight wire conveying a current of electricity the lines of force are circles, concentric with the wire itself as axis, the circles having radii which continually increase without limit. As stated before, the lines of force surrounding an electric current represent the paths which a magnetic north pole would follow if it could move under the influence which is exerted.

The direction of the lines is taken as the direction in which the North pole would move, the south pole being impelled in the opposite direction. Hence, if we had two magnetic poles, a north and south pole, joined by some elastic material which offered almost no resistance to distortion, the magnet thus formed would wrap itself closely around the magnet, the north pole going in one direction, the south pole in the opposite.

From the relation which we already know exists between the force at a point and the number of lines of force at the point, it is evident that if we double the current we double the number of lines of force within a given space; and it is also clear that we may double the current either by doubling the flow of electricity through a single wire, or by placing side by side two wires, each of which conveys the original current. Hence it follows that if we have a coil of wire of a given number of turns, we can produce within the area of the coil a number of lines of force many times as great as for a single turn. If we have a circular wire, the lines of force are still circles very near the wire, but as their radii become larger and larger the circular form is departed from, and near the centre of the coil the lines of force become very much flattened out.

Two wires side by side conveying currents in opposite directions have lines of force around them very much like those shown in Fig. 50. If the currents are in the same direction, the lines of force are as shown in Fig. 51. Now, according to the laws of the action of currents on currents discovered by Ampere, two parallel currents in the same direction attract each other, while two parallel currents in opposite directions repel each other. We can include these two laws in the single statement, originally due to Faraday, that lines of force tend always to shorten themselves. In Fig. 50 we see that the effect of this tendency is to drive the wires farther apart, and in Fig. 51 to draw them more closely together, which is in accordance with what we know experimentally.

In fact, these figures, 50 and 51, are an actual representation of the state of things about two wires carrying currents in the same and in opposite directions. They show the effect which currents have on iron filings, and are reproductions of the positions assumed by particles of iron in the electro-magnetic field.

Let us consider a little more in detail the lines of force around a circular current. Their directions are clearly given in Fig. 52, and we cannot but observe the great similarity between their general form and those due to a small magnet already shown. Indeed, it can be proved mathematically that a cireular current can always, for points not very close to it, be replaced by a very small magnet suspended at its centre. AYe could, therefore, as far as the electrical action is concerned, replace the suspended magnet used in many electrical instruments by a small circular current.

The magnetic force due to a single circular current is, however, in general, quite small, and to increase this there is employed the arrangement known as a solenoid. This is merely a coiled conductor formed by winding a certain length of copper wire over a circular cylinder. Generally the adjacent turns of wire are much closer together than is represented in Fig. 53, and besides it is customary, where intense effects are desired, to use many layers of wire instead of a single layer. The lines of force due to a solenoid are almost identical with those issuing from a long, thin magnet, for when the magnet is very long compared with its diameter the poles are nearly at the ends, and hence the lines of force do not issue from the sides.

In Fig. 54 is represented approximately the direction of the lines of force due to such a solenoid, and the similarity referred to is very apparent.

Clearly, now, if we should place an iron rod within the solenoid these lines of force would pass through the iron and hence magnetize it. Further, on account of the greater conductivity of iron for lines of magnetic force, more lines will pass through the solenoid under these circumstances than if the iron were not present. Hence, by inserting the iron rod we make more lines of force in the space around the solenoid; that is, we created a more *Intense magnetic field*. Again, if the iron is very soft its conductivity is very great, and the magnetic field is stronger than it would have been if we had employed steel or hard iron, but we shall find that in stopping the current its magnetism will almost entirely disappear. If we had used steel there would have been developed, on the contrary, a very strong permanent effect. This is the method which is employed in the making of artificial magnets.

It is found that if we have a large number of turns of wire in the solenoid and send a heavy current through it we can magnetize a rod of steel far more strongly than by any other means, and the time required is also much shortened; indeed, a momentary passage of the current is all that is required.

From what has been said regarding the magnetic action of the electric current it appears that the intensity of the magnetic force within a solenoid, through which electricity is flowing, is measured by the number of turns of wire in the solenoid and by the strength of the current which the coil of wire carries. This is strictly true of the *magnetic force,* but the intensity of magnetism developed thereby does not follow the same law. As long as the magnetizing force is small the magnetism produced in the iron core of the helix or solenoid increases in a regular manner with an increase in the current and number of turns of wire. But after a certain force, as thus measured, is reached the increase in magnetism becomes less marked and tends more and more toward a limiting value.

What this limiting value is depends upon the quality of iron or steel in the helix, and it is much greater for soft iron than for hard iron or steel. When a magnetic body has been magnetized so strongly that a great increase in magnetic force produces only a slight increase in its magnetism, the body is said to be "saturated." *Galvanometers.*—We have learned from Oersted's experiments that a current of electricity in a wire tends in general to deflect magnets near it from their normal position to one at right angles to the current, and the greater the current the greater the angular deflection produced. We could, therefore, construct on this principle an instrument capable of measuring the relative intensity of different currents. Instruments of this kind are now in very general use, and are called *galvanometers* (Fig. 55).

In its most general form a galvanometer is simply a circular coil of wire, fixed by means of a suitable framework in an upright position, and having suspended at its centre a magnet

Fig. 55.—Galvanometer, (Thomson.)

which can rotate about a vertical axis. The magnet itself is generally a small piece of steel strongly magnetized and provided with a pointer and a scale so that its position may be accurately known. A small magnet must be used, so that its poles, in all positions of the needle, may be regarded as sensibly at the centre of the coil, for reasons to be afterward explained, and a pointer is necessary to magnify the angular rotation of the needle.

In the galvanometer the aim is to so arrange the wires that the greatest effect can be secured at a given point with the minimum amount of wire, and to secure this the wires are always arranged in the form of a circle. Generally there are many turns of wire forming the coil of the galvanometer, so that the magnetic force may be great. But the number of turns of wire as well as the size of conductor employed depend upon the currents which are to be measured, and we must choose our galvanometer with this end in view. Hence, if we wish to measure heavy currents we must employ a galvanometer with large wires; first, because its resistance being generally low it does not materially affect the current strength when inserted in the circuit; and, secondly, because it will not be subjected to an undue heating by the current. If we are going to measure very small currents we must have a very sensitive galvanometer, and exceedingly sensitive galvanometers must necessarily have high resistances, because their coils must be composed of fine wire, so that we may have many turns of conductor very close to the suspended needle.

There was at one time a general belief, still held in some cases, that galvanometers of certain kinds were suitable for measuring currents of large "volume " or "great quantity," and that other galvanometers measured the "intensity" of the currents passing through them but not their "volume." This, of course, means nothing. Current, according to definition, is the rate of flow of electricity; that is, it is the quantity of electricity flowing per unit of time; it may be a large current or a small current, but it can never be a quantity current. All galvanometers measure the relative intensity of different currents, and if the instrument has been calibrated so that every reading means a perfectly definite current we can calculate from a given deflection the Quantity of electricity passing through it.

In every form of galvanometer the indications of the needle depend upon the establishment of equilibrium between the magnetic force exerted by the current in the coil and a force in a direction at right angles to this, whether produced by the earth's magnetism, by magnets placed near the instrument, or by springs, etc.

The magnetic force exerted by a coil of wire on a needle placed at its centre is of the nature of what is known in mechanics as a couple; that is, the forces at the two ends of the needle are equal and opposite. Hence, the forces tend to make the needle rotate about its axis, but not to move it as a whole. The needle, therefore, when the current is passing, is deflected from its position at rest, and continues to move until the force

Flg. 56.

of the coil is balanced by the other forces acting, such as the earth's magnetic force. Thus, if the needle occupied normally the position represented by the dotted line *A B,* Fig. 56, and the lines of force due to the coil were shown in direction by the lines *L L,* etc. (which are approximately parallel for a very large coil and a very small needle), then the needle would rotate into the position *A ' B* or *A' B",* depending upon the relative strengths of field due to the coil, and due to the earth.

In the lower figure is seen how the magnetic force of the coil shown by the lines $L\ L$ acts on the needle. The north pole is attracted to the right by the force $N' = Nb$, the south pole to the left by the force $S' = S\ b'$, equal but opposite to N'. These forces, by the well-known laws of resolution applicable to such cases, have each a component along the length of the needle $N\ a$ and $S\ a'$, which, being equal and opposite, neutralize each other; and each a component at right angles to the needle $N\ c$ and $S\ c'$, which are also opposite, but, being parallel, tend to make the needle rotate, as shown.

The forces due to the earth's magnetism, or whatever may be used to direct the needle, are perpendicular to these, and hence the needle will rotate until equilibrium between the two sets of forces is established, and will then more or less quickly come to rest.

When in use, the galvanometer is so placed relatively to the magnetic meridian that its own lines of force and those of the earth are at right angles to each other. This happens when the plane of the coil is directly in the magnetic meridian. It must be remembered that when we speak of the lines of force due to a circular current as being parallel to any given direction, we mean the lines of force *at the centre of the coil,* for a very short distance on either side of the coil's plane. The lines of force are all really curved, but for a very small part of their length, at the coil's centre, they may be regarded as straight, and, if the coil is large, as parallel. (Compare Fig. 52.)

When the coils of the galvanometer are placed in this way, —*i.e.,* parallel to the magnetic meridian,—it may be shown that the current is proportional to the tangent of the' angular deflection of the needle; and when so used the instrument is called a tangent galvanometer.

There is, however, another way in which the galvanometer may be employed: we may move the coils around a vertical axis until the needle which was deflected by the current in the coils is again in the plane of the latter; that is, the current is first allowed to flow and deflect the needle; then, when the needle has come to rest, the coils are turned around until the needle again points to zero. Under these circumstances the current will be proportional to *the sine of* the angle of deflection. Sine galvanometers, since they require a considerable time for adjusting, can only be used when the current is steady.

In many galvanometers there is adopted what is known as the "astatic" arrangement of the needles. This means simply that two equal magnets are so placed with regard to each other that the system is not acted upon by a magnetic field influencing both equally. It is necessary to have two equal magnets, and to place them with their poles in opposite directions, the two magnets being rigidly connected. Such a system of magnets (Fig. 57) suspended anywhere in a uniform magnetic field, *i.e.,* a field which is of the same intensity throughout, will assume one position as well as another; that is, it will be in equilibrium in whatever direction it may point.

To apply this to a galvanometer, one of the magnets is placed inside the coil of wire through which the current to be measured passes, and the other is either entirely outside the coil (Fig. 58) or placed within another coil wound in the opposite direction to the first. In the latter case the magnetic effect of the current is doubled, and the magnetic force of the earth, since it acts equally and in opposite directions on the two magnets, has no effect on the system. Galvanometers of this kind can be constructed with a sensibility so great that they will give a large deflection when there is passed through them a current from a single Daniell cell in series with a resistance of several million ohms.

In order to change the deflection of the galvanometer needle due to a given current we have, in general, to neutralize or increase the strength of the external magnetic field, as well as change its direction. This is usually accomplished by placing near the needle a permanent magnet, which controls its movements, and is, therefore, called a directing magnet. In this way we may vary the angular deflection produced by a given current as much as we please; that is, we can increase the sensibility of the galvanometer or diminish it within very wide limits.

Shunts.—There is still another method of varying the sensibility of a galvanometer, which consists in the employment of the arrangement known as a "shunt." This is simply a coil of wire of a definite resistance joined in parallel with the galvanometer coils (Fig. 59). In the figure G is the galvanometer, to the two terminals of which (-4 and $B)$ are fastened the cntls of the resistance or shunt (i?), the current flowing as indicated by the arrows. The shunt, being in multiple arc with galvanometer, has the effect of diverting a part of the current from the latter, the proportion of this to the whole current being known when the resistances of the shunt and galvanometer coils are given.

According to the statement made on page 37 about circuits joined in parallel, it is evident that we can make any desired proportion of the total current pass through the galvanometer by changing the resistance of the shunt.

Thus, if the resistance of the galvanometer is Rg and that of the shunt i?,, and the difference of potential at the galvanometer terminals is E, then we have for the total current which may also be written hence, the current through the galvanometer being R is that part of the total current which is represented by the fraction.

$R.\ .\ +\ R$ This fraction is called the multiplying power of the shunt. It is evident, therefore, that by making R, very small we can cause only a small part of the current to flow through the galvanometer, and by making it large we can secure the opposite result, thus varying the sensibility of the instrument as much as we please. In general, the resistance of the shunt is so chosen that the current through the galvanometer becomes either , T, or y-jViy of the total current, thus changing the sensibility a thousandfold. For example, if the galvanometer has a resistance of 100 ohms, and we desire to reduce its deflection for a given current C, 10 times, we should join to its terminals a shunt of a resistance equal to llj-ohms, since then the fraction $R.\ R.\ +\ ,$ would be one-

tenth, namely, $J = B'$ io it, $+ wo$
or,
10 S. = B. + 100
9 S, = 100
R. = 11
and so on for any other reduction.

Shunts are of great value in the general use of galvanometers, and nearly all instruments for the measurement of current (and of potential) are provided with shunts as they are, sent out by their manufacturers.

The "ohm" is the *practical* unit of resistance now universally adopted.

Those galvanometers which have heretofore been mentioned are intended almost exclusively for laboratory purposes and are not suited to be moved about. Portable galvanometers are of a more compact form, and the means adopted to keep the needle at its zero position are usually different. In such cases either a very powerful directing magnet is used, so that under its influence the needle is scarcely at all affected by the earth's magnetism, or else the needle is supported by springs which resist its tendency to rotation caused by the current in the coil of the galvanometer. Such instruments are, of course, very liable to derangement; that is, the deflection of the magnet due to a given current gradually changes, because the directing magnet loses gradually its magnetism. This cannot be entirely avoided, but by calibrating the apparatus frequently it is possible to secure sufficient accuracy for all practical purposes.

It is very important to remember that, as long as the conditions remain the same, currents of equal value give identical deflections on the same galvanometer. For, although the currents may be flowing through circuits whose resistances are far from being alike, it is, after all, the final current which we are measuring, and, as equal currents produce equal magnetic fields in the galvanometer coils, the needle must always rotate the same amount for the same current. Even if the galvanometer needle should become weaker the statement still holds true, for, althoiigh it is not as strongly acted upon by the gal-vanometer current when its magnetism is diminished, its motion is also not as strongly resisted by the earth's magnetism, and a balance between the two forces occurs therefore independently of the strength of the magnet, *i.e.,* the needle, itself. Of course this is true only when external conditions are the same; that is, when the magnetic field produced by the earth or by a directing magnet, or the resistance of the spring remains the same; and this we can never be sure of. Indeed, for very accurate work we cannot assume the conditions unchanged even from day to day.

Suppose we have an ordinary Daniell cell joined in circuit with a galvanometer whose resistance, together with that of the connecting wires, is one "ohm." Since the resistance of the cell itself is four ohms, approximately, the current will be —1— = of the unit of current. Instead of speaking of units of current, etc., let us call the unit resistance one ohm, the unit current one ampere, and the unit electro-motive force one volt. Then the above current will be ampere. Suppose, now, we had fifty cells of this kind joined in series, the current in this case would be 8ft;that is, 50 volts divided by 200 ohms (= 50 X 4 '+ 1), equal to of an ampere, nearly; hence the galvanometer deflection would not be *very* different in the two cases, although we have increased the electro-motive force fifty times. The reason is that, notwithstanding the large increase in elcctro-motiv'e force, we have increased the total resistance of the circuit nearly in the same proportion, since the cells make up almost the entire resistance themselves.

But, suppose the galvanometer had a resistance of 10,000 ohms, then one cell would give a current of only ij ampere, while fifty cells would give a current of jV , xa xS almost fifty times as great. In this case the current would be increased approximately in proportion to the number of cells, for now the cells compose a small part of the total resistance.

Galvanometers which are direct-reading are generally called ampere, or mill-ampere, meters, or more simply ammeters, the name being taken from the practical unit of current called the ampere. (See page 119.) *Potential Galvanometers, or Voltmeters.*—Galvanometers are used not only to measure currents, but are also employed to measure differences of potential. The principal of construction is, however, the same, since the difference of potential is indicated by the *current* passing through the galvanometer, and about the measurement of this we have already learned.

In the use of the instrument for this purpose the two terminals are joined to the points whose potential we desire to measure, and the galvanometer coils are therefore in multiple arc with the conductor, along which there exists the difference of potential referred to. Thus, in Fig. 61, $A B$ is the conductor through which is flowing the current, and along which at the points $Di\ D2$ are the potentials I'j $V2$ respectively. The galvanometer wires are joined to the points $Du\ Dx\ G$ being the potential galvanometer. If Rc is the resistance of the conductor between the points Dv and D and Ru the resistance of the galvanometer, we know from page 71 that the currents through them will be, respectively, and the whole current will be the sum of these, or

By inserting in parallel arc the galvanometer between the points and F2 we have diminished the total resistance between these points, since the current has two paths in which it can flow. If the galvanometer is not joined, the whole current, instead of dividing itself between Rc and lia will remain in the wire Rc. Hence, the difference of potential is less when the galvanometer is joined to the points than it was before. When the galvanometer is out of circuit the current in the main wire $A B$ is

When the galvanometer is in circuit it is as before given, where

Now, in the first case we have r, _ $ra = C\ R0$ in the second case, r, — $Va = C\ r$ but r is less than Rc and hence the difference of potential is less in the second case than in the first. But we desire to know the difference of potential exactly under these circumstances, hence we must see that the introduction of the galvanometer causes the smallest possible error.

From the above equation we see that $F_j — V_2$ will be. more and more nearly the same in the two cases, the more nearly equal are R_c and r; that is to say, the larger we make R_g. If the latter is exceedingly large, then - is exceedingly small, so that we can finally neglect it, and instead of writing = -+ -
r Rc B9
we can write, approximately, i= i_ rRB which is the required condition. Hence, in order to use a galvanometer to measure differences of potential, it is very necessary that its resistance be high. We must, in other words, make its resistance so high that the current which may flow through it will not materially disturb the difference of potential existing at the points to which it is to be joined.

Method of Reading Galvanometer Deflections.—" The reading of galvanometer deflections requires considerable method in order that accurate results may be obtained in making measurements. Let A and B (Figs. 62, 63, 64, 65) be two contiguous division marks on the galvanometer scale. Now, by observation we can always determine without difficulty whether the pointer lies exactly over A or over B, or whether it lies exactly midway between the two; and further, if it does not occupy either of these exact positions, we can judge without difficulty whether it lies nearest to A or to B. This is equivalent to saying that we can be certain of the magnitude of the deflection within a quarter of a degree. Thus, supposing the pointer stood between A and B, but nearer to A than to B, then we should call the deflection A, and, supposing the deflection was actually *very m*
Deflection = A Deflection =A Deflection = *M* A Deflection =A
Fig. 62. Fig. 63. Fig. 64. Fig. 63.
nearly equal to A, then A would be a quarter of a division, or a degree too much; if, on the other hand, the deflection was *very* nearly equal to A, then A would be a quarter of a division, or a degree too little. In one case the error would be a plus one, and in the other a minus one, but in either case its *maximum* value would be only. We have, in fact, the rule that, if A be the smaller of the contiguous deflections A and B, then when the pointer is exactly over A the deflection should be called 'A;' if nearer to A than to B, it should be called 'A;' if exactly midway between A and B, it should be called '-4£;' and lastly, if the pointer is nearer to B than to A, then the deflection should be called '-4;' thus, for example, if B and A (Figs. 62, 63, 64, 65) were the 57 and 58 division marks respectively on the scale, then, in case 1 the deflection would be taken as 57, in case 2 the deflection would be taken as 57, and again, in cases 3 and 4, the deflections would be taken as 57i and 57 respectively." Hand-book Electrical Testing, Kenipe, p. 41.

By keeping to these instructions, then, we can be certain of the magnitude of a deflection within of a division or degree.

Dynamometers.—According to Ampere's laws of the mutual action of currents (page G3), we know that currents which are parallel and in the same direction attract each other, and we can prove that this attraction is greater the greater the currents and the closer together the conductors carrying them. This is, then, another phenomenon which we could make use of for the measurement of currents. Instruments constructed on this principle, *i.e.*, depending for their action on the mutual force existing between wires conveying electric currents, are called dynamometers (Fig. 66). Such instruments possess this important advantage over galvanometers: they are not subject to the errors resulting from the variable magnetization of directing magnets, etc., and the changes in the earth's field.

Dynamometers consist essentially of two coils of wire, placed at right angles to each other, one of which is movable and one fixed (Figs. 67, 68, and 69). The movable coil, A, is generally quite small compared with the fixed coil, B, and is suspended within this by means of two very thin and parallel wires, W, forming what is called a *bifilar* suspension. These wires, through which the current is led to the suspended coil, must be thin and offer but little resistance to torsion. When heavier currents are to be measured, the ends of the suspended coil are carried to a pair of mercury cups, C C (Fig. 69), placed beneath, and the circuit is completed through these. In this case the wires, A, or, better, silk fibres, making the suspension, have nothing to do with the current.

When the current is passed through both coils their mutual electro-magnetic action tends to make them become parallel, the rotational effort being greater the greater the current. The angular movement thereby resulting is resisted by the bifilar suspension itself, which tends to keep the coils perpendicular to each other. Hence, during the passage of the current the movable coil will swing around until a balance between the two forces is effected, and from the deflection we can, knowing the number of turns of wire on the two coils, their mean radius, etc., calculate at once the current.

The wires or silk threads of the suspended coil are attached to a graduated circle, which can be moved about a vertical axis, and which serves to adjust the coil to any desired position. In the use of the instrument it is customary to move the circle, C (Fig. 70), to which are attached the threads (the current being supposed to flow), until the deflected coil is brought back to its zero position; that is, until it is again peipendicular to the fixed coil surrounding it (not shown in Fig. 70). This, as in the employment of the sine galvanometer, cannot be done unless the currents are so steady that they do not change while the adjustment is being made. We can, however, provide the suspended coil with a divided circle and index, and thus determine at once the angular deflection due to the current which is passing, and this method is also frequently adopted, especially when it becomes necessary to make rapid measurements.

The electro-dynamometer has a wider range of usefulness than any galvanometer, however made, because it can be applied to the measurement of alternating currents, *i.e.*, alternating currents with many alternations per second.

Galvanometers are entirely unsuited for this very r important kind of work, the reason being that, as the currents are alternately plus and minus, —that is, first in one direction and then in the opposite,—the needle is rapidly impelled first to one side and then to the other, with the final result that it remains at rest. If the period of the current is large compared with the time of vibration of the needle, the latter will swing backward and forward, but will not take up any definite position. In the latter case the galvanometer needle would follow the current and swing from side to side, but would, of course, give no permanent deflection.

The formula for the Weber electro-dynamometer, in which there are two fixed coils and one or two—in the latter case rigidly connected—suspended coils, is $C = $ -'- $tn\&$
A $ig\ T'$
$C = -A\sin t$

In this, C Is the current to be measured, T is the time of vibration of the suspended coil, A its moment of inertia as suspended, » the angular deflection of the coil, and G and g constants of the two sets of coils (best determined by careful measurement). As the instrument is sent out by the manufacturer, we have only to multiply the *square root* of the angle by a constant, determined beforehand, in order to find the current.

In the dynamometer the change of direction of the current has no effect, because it is changed in both coils at the same time. Hence, if, when the current is flowing in one direction, the suspended coil is driven to the right, say; then, when the current is reversed, the deflection will still be in the same direction, because the lines of force due to *both coils* have been reversed.

The phenomenon is exactly the same as would occur if we could reverse the magnetism of the needle of a galvanometer every time the current changed its direction. Thus, in Fig. 71, suppose, with the current in the direction indicated, the north pole of the needle turns to the right. Now (Fig. 72), suppose when the current changes its direction we reverse the poles of the magnet, A making the right-hand side a south pole and the left-hand side a north pole. The lines of force are in the opposite direction, as shown, and the north pole will follow them; but, the needle's magnetism having been also reversed, it is already in the direction of the lines of force, and hence does not move.

Now, in a dynamometer, instead of a magnetic needle to be acted upon, we have a coil of wire, and the direction of the lines of force of this coil are really changed every time the direction of the current is changed. Hence, since the current changes its direction simultaneously in both coils, we have the same effect as if the current remained perfectly constant.

But it must be remembered that we have all along supposed that the time required for the current to change from a positive to a negative value was very small compared with the time of vibration of the suspended coil of the dynamometer. If they are nearly equal the coil will swing around every time the current changes from plus to minus, and will therefore be rendered utterly useless for measurements.

However, this seldom occurs in practice, since the period of most alternating currents is a very small fraction of a second.

According to Ampere's laws, the mutual action between two currents is proportional to the strength of the currents multiplied together. Hence, we may express the action of the dynamometer by saying that its deflections are proportional to the products, or squares of currents, and therefore it is immaterial whether the currents are both plus or minus (since the *product* of two *negative* quantities gives a pasture result), provided they are both plus or minus at the *same time.*

Again, we have found that the energy of a current is measured by the square of its intensity. Consequently, since the dynamometer in reality measures the square of the current its indications are proportional to the *energy* of the current passing through it. In order to determine the current itself it is necessary to take the square root of the angular deflection (or its sine) of the suspended coil.

Induction of Electric Currents.—Consider the case of a closed metallic circuit (Fig. 73), including a galvanometer, and a magnet near it. Suppose, now, that the magnet is suddenly pulled away from the wire to a distance, and, after a few minutes, as suddenly brought back to its first position. We shall observe that the It is usual to refer to a complete circuit—that is, a circuit which is continuous throughout —as a "*closed*" circuit, and a circuit which is interrupted at any point as an "*open*" or, some times, a broken circuit. galvanometer needle will swing to one side when the magnet is being withdrawn, and then swing through the same angle on the other side when the magnet is being carried near to the coil. This effect is not due to any direct action of the large magnet on the galvanometer needle, for the same thing happens when the galvanometer is so far away that it cannot be so influenced; and the phenomenon does *not* take place if the metallic circuit is broken at any point. Hence, by the movement of a magnet near a conductor we can produce a current in the conductor, and a current so produced is called a *current of induction,* or an *induced current.*

If, instead of removing the magnet to a distance, we had rotated it or changed its position in any way, supposing it to be near the wire $A\ B$ (Fig. 74), similar though probably less-marked effects would have been noticed. Further, if instead of a magnet we had employed another circuit, $C\ D$ (Fig. 74), through which a current was flowing *(M* being a battery), we would have produced a current in the circuit $A\ D$ every time the circuits changed their relative positions, as well as every time the intensity of the current in $C\ D$ was changed. With Fig. 74.

the latter arrangement we would make the galvanometer needle swing through the same angle, whether we removed *instantaneously* the circuit *CDs.* great distance or broke the circuit completely, so that the current flowing through it would be suddenly stopped.

Now, we know that the circle of wire near the magnet surrounds, in a given position, a certain number of lines of force due to the magnet. Again, if the circuits *A B* and *C D* are parallel and close together, the former has passing through it a large number of the lines of magnetic force resulting from the current.in *CD*. By changing the relative positions of the magnet and the circuit *A B,* or of the two circuits *A B* and *C D,* we alter the number of lines of force passing through the circuit *A B;* that is, we alter the "induction," as it is called, through it.

These phenomena, and many others of a similar kind, can be included under the one general law,—when the induction through a metallic circuit is changed it becomes the seat of an electro-motive force, the magnitude of which is proportional to the rate of change of induction. Instead of saying rate of change of induction, it is sometimes convenient to speak of rate of cutting lines of magnetic force, the latter statement expressing the idea in a more popular but less accurate way. Hence, when a conductor cuts across lines of magnetic force (and this may happen either when the conductor itself moves or the lines of force move), there is an electro-motive force set up in the conductor which will give rise to an electric current if the circuit is complete so that a current can flow. The direction of the electro-motive force depends both upon the direction of the lines of force and the direction of movement of the conductor. If, for instance, the conductor *A B,* Fig. 75 (X *L,* etc., being lines of magnetic force), moving downward, *i.e.,* perpendicularly to plane of paper, has set up in it an electro-motive force, as indicated by the arrow from *A* to *B,* then on moving it upward the electro-motive force would act in the direction from *B* to *A.* Or, if the lines of force were in the opposite direction, then a downward movement of *A B* would correspond with an upward movement in the former case.

The question of induction of magnets on currents and of currents on currents included under the name *electro-magnetic induction* has been very fully investigated by Faraday. He found that the electro-motive force produced by the movement of a conductor across lines of magnetic force was independent of the nature of the conductor, and of its thickness in the direction of the lines of force. Thus, a bar of steel an inch thick and a foot long would have induced in it, by being carried across a magnetic field, the same electro-motive force as a bar of copper two inches thick, but also a foot long, both moving with the same velocity. The currents in the two cases, supposing the. ends of the bar to be joined by similar wires, might be very different, notwithstanding the equality in the electro-motive forces, because the currents depend upon the *total resistances* of the circuits.

Since the electro-motive force induced in a wire by its movement in a magnetic field is equal to the rate of cutting lines of force, it is clear that it will be greatest for a given velocity when the conductor moves perpendicularly to the lines of force, and will be less and less the more oblique the direction of motion. If we increase the slant so that the conductor moves directly along the lines of force there is no effect at all produced. This is evident from Fig. 76, where it is shown how much nearer together are the lines of force if we proceed in the direction *A B* than if we go along *A C.*

Again, we can increase the induced electro-motive force as much as we please by making the conductor consist of a large number of turns of wire, because, since each turn of wire cuts across the lines of force independently, each wire has the same electro-motive force produced in it, and we have the effect of all added together. Thus, if we have a circle of one turn of wire and another of three turns, then the electro-motive force produced in the latter, by causing the same change of induction to take place through both coils, will be three times that produced in the former.

If we move nearer together two parallel circles facing each other, in each of which a current is flowing,—say in the same direction,—the motion will be aided, as we know by the mutual attraction of the circles. (See page 62.) At the same time the induction through each of the circles changes; that is, the number of lines of force included by them is varied by the movement; therefore, each circle must become independently the seat of an electro-motive force which will augment or diminish the original electro-motive force present according to its direction.

These phenomena" have been carefully studied by Lenz, who announced the law that the induced currents are always in such directions that they tend, by their electro-magnetic action, to resist the change which produced them. In the case cited above the circuits attract each other, having currents in the same direction; hence, the induced electro-motive forces must be such as to diminish the attraction, and, therefore, in the opposite direction to the original electro-motive forces. The total electro-motive force being the difference between the two others in opposite directions (the original and the induced), and being, therefore, diminished, has the result of reducing the original current, this diminution continuing as long as the motion is kept up.

We can, by the application of Lenz's law, determine in every case the direction of the induced electro-motive force resulting from the action of magnets on currents, and of the latter on themselves.

Faraday's and Lenz's laws also offer an explanation of the oft-observed phenomenon, that, when a current is made, there is but a very small spark ensuing, whereas, when it is broken, the spark is very noticeable, especially so when the circuit contains a coil of wire wound over a rod of soft iron. The reason is this: When the current begins to flow through a coil, the coil becomes at once surrounded by lines of force, which, in expanding outward, must necessarily pass through the wires of the coil themselves. But this they cannot do without inducing electro-motive forces all along the coil, and, according to Lenz's law, the directions of the induced electro-motive forces are such as to resist the change by which they are caused. Hence, they must be opposed to the electro-motive force of the source, so that at the instant of contact the total electro-motive force in the circuit is small, and there is consequently scarcely any spark. On breaking the circuit, however, the lines of force collapse suddenly and again pass through the wires. But the electro-motive force set up this time must aid the electro-motive force of the source, since its direction must be such as to resist the change, *i.e.*, the stopping of the current. Consequently, at the moment of breaking the circuit the electro-motive force is comparatively high, being the sum, instead of the difference, of the induced electro-motive force and that of the source; and hence the current tends to leap across the break in the form of a spark.

The spark is diminished on closing and increased on breaking the circuit by the presence of an iron rod in a coil of wire included in the circuit, because more lines of force are formed in this case, as we have already found. (See page 64.)

The lines of force around any circuit due to its own current are called the "self-induction " of the circuit; hence the greater the self-induction the greater the spark-length.

Induction Coils.—The rapid passage of lines of magnetic force across a conductor resulting in the production of an induced electro-motive force in the metal has a practical application, and a very important one, in the induction coil, better known as the "Ruhmkorff Induction Apparatus."

The Ruhmkorff coil (Figs. 77 and 78) consists, in its usual form, of an electromagnet, e, the magnetizing current flowing through the wire A *(B* being the battery), surrounded by a number of turns of, generally finer, wire, *a a.* The circuits are entirely independent, having no metallic connection whatever with each other, and the circuit, *A A,* which conveys the magnetizing current around the mass of iron inside it, *c b,* is called the *primar;/* circuit, while the circuit a a is called the *secondary.* Sometimes the coils are so arranged that one can slide over the other so as to completely surround it, or can be moved off to a considerable distance, as in Fig. 79. In order to render

FIG. 77.—RtTHMKOKFP INDUCTION *COTL.* the action between the coils susceptible of a still greater variation the secondary coil is olten pivoted so that its axis may be a prolongation of that of the primary coil, or may make any desired angle in a horizontal plane with this. As a rule, the primary coil is made of quite thick wire, and consists of a comparatively small number of turns; the secondary, however, is of much finer wire and has a large number of turns. In the circuit of the primary coil there is inserted one or more cells of a battery, *B* (Fig. 80), and it includes also a contact-breaker, A". The latter is simply a small vibrating knob of iron, *H,* which is moved backward by the action of a spring, *S,* and when released strikes against the core of the electro-magnet. Being iron it is attracted by the iron core, C, where this is magnetized, and is pulled away by its spring when the core is demagnetized, since the core then loses its attractive influence. The object of the vibrating lever, *K,* is to periodically stop the primary current, which it does by breaking contact at some point, *K,* in the circuit. Such an arrangement is on this account generally called a "make and break."

The mode of action of the coil is as follows: The lever *L* is first pulled back so that the contact is made at /l'and the current allowed to flow through the primary circuit. The current thus flowing magnetizes the iron core, and this pulls the piece of soft iron on c the lever over until it touches the core. But at this moment contact at *K* is broken so that the current stops, the core loses its magnetism, and the little iron armature is again drawn backward by the action of the spring, *S.* As it moves backward it makes contact at *K* again, the current flows once more, and the same series of phenomena is repeated. This making and breaking of the primary current can be made to take place with any degree of rapidity desired by changing the period of the swinging lever.

Now, every time the current is made, lines of force shoot outward from the coil and cut across the wires of the secondary circuit. Hence (page 84), the secondary circuit becomes the seat of an electro-motive force, first in one direction, then in the other, according as the lines of force are moving inward or outward. It is thus an alternating electro-motive force. The magnitude of this depends upon the number of turns of wire in the secondary coil, and upon the number of lines of force sent outward by the primarv circuit in the unit time; that is, it depends upon the rate of change of induction through the secondary' coil.

The electro-motive force thus induced in the secondary circuit may be many times as great as that existing in the primary coil. Indeed, it is an easy matter to increase it from the electro-motive force of a single cell to that of several thousand cells; all that is necessary is to have a large number of turns of wire in the secondary circuit, and to make the lines of force move very quickly. The latter is secured in two ways: first, by making the armature vibrate quickly, and, secondly, by employing for the iron core of the primary circuit a bundle of soft-iron wires instead of a solid iron rod. The bundle of wires is much more rapidly magnetized and demagnetized than a solid core would be, and we have an explanation of this in the known relations existing between the direction of lines of force and the direction of the resulting currents. For, the same lines of force which move inward and outward and thus produce electro-motive forces in the secondary circuit tend to give rise to currents in the mass of the iron core itself. Thus, every time we have an electro-motive force in a given direction produced in the secondary circuit we have an electro-motive force in the same direction in the iron core. Now, by Lenz's law these electro-motive forces tend to produce currents in such directions that they resist the changes by which they are caused. Therefore, when a piece of iron is magnetized or demagnetized by electro-magnetic action the currents induced in its own substance are in such directions as to diminish for the time being the magnetization and also the demagnetization. But if we so subdivide the magnet that these currents cannot flow freely in it we make the iron capable of assuming its final state so much the more rapidly. This is the province of the bundle of iron wires, their lengths being perpendicular to the directions in which the currents tend to circulate.

We must not suppose, because the electro-motive force induced in the secondary circuit is so many times as great as that in the primary, that we have, by this means, increased the *energy* of the currents. In reality, under the most favorable circumstances, the efficiency of the usual Ruhmkorff coil is about 65 to 70 per cent.

Although we have a very high electro-motive force induced in the secondary circuit, the current in this is very small, and we know that the energy of a current depends not upon the electromotive force, nor upon current-intensity alone, but upon the product of these two. So in the induction coil, if we should actually measure the energy in the secondary wires we should find it always less than three-fourths that of the primary. In most cases, 25 per cent, at least of the energy of the primary current is lost, and, although it is converted into some other form of energy (mostly heat), it is not available in the secondary circuit.

Only a small electro-motive force is required to maintain the current in the primary circuit, one or two cells being ordinarily sufficient. Nevertheless, an account of the way in which its wires are coiled over a mass of iron (page 64) the electromotive force due to its own self-induction may be considerable, and a spark may pass between the points of the contact breaker (7s.") from this circumstance. In this way the metal surfaces become worn away, or corroded, so that finally a good contact cannot be made. To avoid such action, as far as possible, the points at which the circuit is opened and closed are sometimes immersed in alcohol, which greatly lessens the difficulty. One pole is connected with a cup containing some mercury, covered over with alcohol, while the other pole is a rod which makes contact by dipping into the mercury, and in this way the destructive sparking is almost completely avoided.

As stated before, the electro-motive force of the secondary coil (a, Fig. 78), in many kinds of induction apparatus, is regulated by varying the distance and angular position of the secondary coil with regard to the primary. It is very easy to see that, as a consequence, the number of lines of force passing through the secondary coil will be subjected to great changes. It is, however, an error to suppose that the number is proportional to the distance between the coils; that is, that the electro-motive force will be twice as great, say, when the distance between the coils is halved. As a matter of fact, so long as one coil surrounds the other, the changes in the electro-motive force induced in the secondary are nearly proportional to the distance between the centres of the coils. But when the secondary coil has moved so far over the primary that the two coils are end for end, the effect becomes suddenly very much reduced. Figure 81 represents the relation between the electro-motive force of the secondary coil, and the distance between it and the primary, for an ordinary Du Bois-Rcymond coil, supposing the same current to flow always through the latter.

On the horizontal line are measured the distances between the coils, and along the vertical line the corresponding electromotive forces produced in the secondary. At *0* the one coil completely surrounded the other; at about *D* the secondary has been moved so far over the primary that they are end for end. The small change in the electro-motive force after this point is reached is clearly shown in the figure, which is taken from a test of a Du Bois-Reymond apparatus. The reason of this is, that the lines of force due to the primary current do not extend outward very far from the ends of the magnet core, but the greater number proceed from pole to pole in the shortest possible paths. At any rate, only a lew lines extend outward to a very great distance from the magnet core. Hence, after the coils have become actually separated, *i.e.,* after they are placed end for end, there are but slight differences in the electromotive forces produced in the secondary coil for greater distances between them.

Another method of regulation, one used very extensively in small induction coils made for medical purposes, consists in the employment of a copper or brass cylinder which is capable of sliding over the iron core of the primary coil. In Fig. 82, *M* is the soft-iron core of the primary circuit, P, surrounding which is the metal cylinder, C, which can be pulled out as far as desired, and S is the secondary circuit of fine wire. The object' of the metal cylinder is to shield the iron core from the magnetic influence of the current in the primary circuit, which it does by preventing the lines of force from reaching the iron. They are retarded in their movements, in their sudden expansion and collapse, by the currents which they themselves produce in the copper cylinder as they tend to pass through it, and, therefore, do not reaoh the iron beneath. Hence, by varying the position of the copper "damper," as it may very appropriately be called, we can shield as much of the iron as we please from magnetic influence, and thus reduce the number of lines of force passing through the secondary circuit at will. When the shield is pushed in as far as possible, the iron core is scarcely at all magnetized; the apparatus has virtually become an induction coil *without* an iron core, and it therefore gives low electromotive forces.

In speaking of the induction coil, it may not be out of place to refer to the inaccurate statements sometimes made regarding the nature of the secondary current,—statements which are often utterly absurd. It is claimed, for instance, that the character of the secondary current depends upon the size of wire used in the secondary winding, apparently irrespective of any change in the electromotive force itself. A winding of thick wire is supposed to have some physiological influence which a coil of thin wire could never exert, etc.

CHAPTER III.

Batteries And Cells. *Primary Batteries.*—Although until recent years the primary hattery has been the only available source of electricity (leaving out of consideration electro-static machines and thermo-electric apparatus), there have been made very *i'ew* improvements of any importance since the first battery came into use. There are many kinds of primary batteries, but the principle of all is the same, and it depends in every case upon the establishment of an electro-motive force at the surface of separation of two metals, or of a metal and a fluid.

The question as to the seat of electromotive force in a battery is still in an unsettled condition. It is claimed by some that the difference of potential is established by the mere contact of dissimilar substances; others look toward chemical action for an explanation, and perhaps the majority believe that both chemical action and contact are necessarily concerned in the phenomenon.

Be that as it may, it is easy to prove that when a metal is plunged into a fluid which is capable of chemically attacking it, a difference of potential is set up between the metal and the fluid. The extent of this difference depends upon the nature of the metal and of the fluid, but is constant, at a given temperature, for the same substances.

Primary batteries may very conveniently be divided into two groups, called respectively one-fluid and two-fluid batteries.

One-fluid *Batteries.*—Cells containing a single fluid—in general, dilute sulphuric acid—are made by dipping two different metals into the liquid, the metals being usually in the form of flat or cylindrical plates, and being provided with binding posts to which the circuit wires may be attached.

It has been stated that if we immerse a plate of zinc and a plate of copper into water containing a little sulphuric acid (Fig. 84), there is set up a difference of potential between the metals. This difference of potential acts, outside the cell, from the copper to the zinc; that is to say, the copper is the positive electrode, and the zinc the negative. Outside the battery, therefore, the current flows from the copper to the zinc, but inside the cell it flows from the zinc to the copper. This is z c expressed by saying that the electro-motive force between the zinc and the dilute acid is greater than that between the copper and acid, which causes the tendency of a current in the direction from zinc to copper through the acid. The electromotive force of the cell is, consequently, the difference of potential between the zinc and copper. The chemical actions which take place in a cell of this kind are, first, the formation of sulphate of zinc, by the action of the acid on the negative plate, and, nwondly, the liberation of hydrogen gas at the positive plate. Thus, the zinc is continually being converted into sulphate of zinc, and this loss is—leaving out local actions—proportioned to S,n whole quantity of electricity which has passed through the o. ih

The internal resistance of most one-fluid batteries is very high, and the current which can be obtained from them is necessarily limited thereby. In order to diminish this resistance as much as possible, the zinc and copper plates are sometimes arranged in the form of a spiral, so as to present a very large surface for the passage of the current (Fig. 85). Thus, by allowing the spirals to be separated by only a small interval, the internal resistance can be made as small as we please. The *electro-motive force* of the battery is independent of the size of the plates and of their distance apart, since it depends solely on the nature of the metals used, and their temperature. The only end which can be attained by the employment of large plates is a corresponding reduction in the internal resistance of the battery, on which depends the intensity of the current which the battery can furnish. It is nearly always an advantage to have a battery with a low internal resistance, if this can be secured without detriment to other important features of a good cell.

There are serious objections to almost all one-fluid cells; they are as follow: *First,* the gradual dilution of the acid solution, which renders it less and less capable of acting on the zinc plate; *second!;/,* the increase of internal resistance due to this extreme dilution of the acid; *thirdly,* the deposition of zinc from the solution of zinc sulphate, or other salt, on the copper plate, which tends to diminish the effective electro-motive force of the plates, inasmuch as, instead of having a circuit made up of *zinc — acid — copper,* we have finally an almost inert circuit, *zinc — acid — zinc* (practically two plates of the same metal, instead of different metals); and, *fourthly,* the 'polarization' of the copper plate, as it is called." This polarization is simply the formation of a film of hydrogen on the copper plate, which not only increases the internal resistance of the cell (hydrogen being comparatively a poor conductor), but also tends to

The res'stance of a galvanic cell is called its internal *raistance.* Th's is the resistance which is opposed to the flow of the current through the cell itself, *i. e.,* from one pole, or electrode, to the other, diminish its electro-motive force. The reason of this is that the electromotive force of copper-hydrogen is in the same direction as that of copper-sulphuric acid, and both being opposite to zinc-sulphuric acid the total electro-motive force is diminished by this amount. All these things make most cells of the onefluid type very unreliable, for not only is their electro-motive force variable, but also, as shown, their internal resistance, both of which should be as constant as possible.

These difficulties have been, to a great extent, overcome in some recent one-fluid cells, which will be described later. (Seepage 102, Fig. 91.) *Two-fluid Batteries.*—Many of the obstacles presented in the use of one-fluid batteries are overcome by replacing the single fluid by two fluids. In these batteries two solutions are employed, and they are separated from each other either by taking advantage of their different specific gravities or by means of porous earthenware vessels.

Daniell Cell.—Probably the best-known type of the twofluid cell is that called the Daniell Element (Fig. 86). In this cell the fluids are a saturated solution of sulphate of copper, CS, and a semi-saturated solution of sulphate of zinc, ZS. In the copper-sulphate solution is placed a sheet of metallic copper, C, and in the zinc-sulphate solution a mass of zinc, Z, these two metals forming the electrodes of the cell. The general forms in which these cells are made are shown in Figs. 87 and 88. The only real difference between the various styles are the methods of keeping the solutions separated. This is done in Fig. 86 by means of an earthenware vessel, P, which, being porous, does not offer a very great resistance to the current, yet prevents to a great extent the mixture of the solutions by diffusion. In all the figures Z is the zinc electrode, generally in the form of a ring, provided with three or four projections, which extend outside the rim of the glass jar and keep it in place. G is the copper electrode marked +, consisting simply of a copper plate or disk having fastened to it an insulated copper wire, which extends upward beyond the liquid in the cell. This wire is covered with some insulating material, such as gutta-percha, which prevents the wire itself from coming in contact with the zinc-sulphate solution.

In the bottom of the cell and surrounding the copper plate is the copper-sulphate solution, CS, which is kept in a saturated condition by being in contact with some crystals of the salt, which dissolve as the solution becomes weaker. In Fig. 86 the coppersulphate solution is kept within the porous vessel, and outside this is the zinc-sulphate solution; but in the other two figures (Figs. 87 and 88) the zinc-sulphate solution, having a smaller specific gravity than the copper-sulphate solution, floats on the top of this without the aid of a separating medium or diaphragm. In the figures, B is the binding-post to which the circuit wires may be attached.

Fig. 88 is intended to show a form of *Daniell cell* which is very convenient for testing purposes, especially when many cells are required. It is made of an ordinary drinking-glass, and is, therefore, much smaller than the usual cell. It is, however, in all other respects identical with those described.

In general, the resistance of these cells is quite high, amounting to about five ohms. It can, however, be diminished indefinitely, just as in the case of one-fluid cells, by using very large metal plates and placing them very close together.

The chemical actions going on in the Daniell cell are as follow: The zinc plate becomes oxidized, and, under the action of the sulphuric acid, is gradually converted into sulphate of zinc. The sulphate of copper is decomposed into oxide of copper, which breaks up further, so that in the end copper is deposited on the copper plate. This, therefore, grows larger at the expense of the copper-sulphate solution, which would thus become weaker were it not for the presence of the crystals of salt. At both plates gases are formed, in consequence of the action of the sulphuric acid on zinc at one electrode (the negative), and of the breaking down of the copper sulphate into H2SO, (sulphuric acid), copper and oxygen at the other.

But oxygen and hydrogen are separated out from the water at the negative and positive electrodes respectively, and the hydrogen thus formed combines with the oxygen from the oxide of copper, and hence forms water back again, the same thing taking place at the zinc pole. Thus, no free gas appears at either electrode, and the phenomenon known as polarization, which consists in the deposition of gases on the surfaces of the metallic plates, and which is so grave an objection to the one-fluid battery, is thereby avoided. If the solutions are kept constant, and the plates carefully looked after, the Daniell cell will give a practically constant electro-motive force for very long periods. But it requires much attention.

Grove Cell.—Another very well known cell, especially so in its variously modified forms, is that called the Grove cell (Fig. 89).

In this cell (Fig. 90) the two active fluids are diluted sulphuric and nitric acids, S and 2V, and the metals immersed in them are respectively zinc and platinum, Z and P.

The acids are separated by means of a porous cup, C, and the general form of the battery is shown in Figs. 90 and 91. Here Z represents the zinc plate, a circular cylinder having a longitudinal slit along its whole length in order to allow the sulphuric acid, S, in which it is immersed to circulate freely on both sides of it. C is the porous cup separating the nitric acid, N, within it from the sulphuric acid, S, outside, and P is the platinum electrode, which is simply a rod of platinum provided with a binding-post.

The reactions which take place in this cell are the conversion of zinc into sulphate of zinc and the combination of the hydrogen formed at the negative pole—the platinum bar—with nitric acid to form water and hyponitric acid. In consequence, the evolution of nitrous fumes, in large quantities, accompanies the use of this style of battery, because only a part of the gases p liberated are absorbed by the water.

The platinum is not attacked by the acid, and will, therefore, last indefinitely. But the zinc is likely to be rapidly consumed unless carefully amalgamated.

The value of the Grove cell consists in its low internal resistance (which in cells of ordinary size is less than a quarter of an ohm) and its high electro-motive force (which under favorable conditions is nearly two volts). The nitrous fumes given off during the action of the cell, which are not only disagreeable but dangerous, are the objection to its use. Furthermore, although the electro-motive force is high under favorable circumstances, it diminishes greatly when the concentration of the acids falls below a certain value.

Bunsen Cell.—In the Bunsen cell the platinum electrode is replaced by a stick of carbon, otherwise the Bunsen and Grove elements are exactly alike in their arrangement. But the electromotive force of the Bunsen cell is somewhat greater than that of the Grove, an advantage which is, however, counterbalanced by its higher internal resistance.

Chromate of Potash Cell.—Another very similar cell is quite extensively employed in place of the preceding, because it is free ' from the objectionable nitrous fumes referred to. In this cell (called the bi-chromatc element) instead of nitric acid a solution of chromic acid—formed previously by the action of sulphuric acid on potassium chromate—is used in the porous cup, and into v this is placed the carbon rod. Moreover, 7 J the sulphuric acid is frequently replaced by I a saturated solution of common salt. This cell has also an electro-motive force of about two volts,— more accurately, 1.87 volts. *Chloride of Silver Battery.*—A battery which gives a practically constant electromotive force during a large number of hours' use is a modification of the chloride of silver cell brought into prominence by De la Rue some years since. The cells as now manufactured in this country are represented in Fig. 91. Here G is a glass vessel about three-quarters of an inch in diameter and two or three inches long, provided with a double stopper, the lower one, 0, being composed of resin and resin-oil, and the upper, S, of plaster of Paris. The vessel contains a paste made of flour and sulphate of zinc, into which dip the metal electrodes. These are rods or plates of zinc, Z, there being two of these, and between them is a rod of chloride of silver, A. A silver wire is attached to the silver-chloride electrode, and passes out through the stopper.

To the zinc electrodes are fastened copper wires, carried through the stopper in the same manner. These cells have an electro-motive force of almost exactly one volt, and are said to remain constant for very long periods.

91 has an internal resistance of about three or four ohms others are constructed with larger plates having a resistance of

The cell shown in Fig. but

something like half an ohm. Through a proper external resistance such cells are able to furnish currents of sufficient intensity to be applicable to almost any variety of medical practice.

Flg. 93.

Figs. 92 and 93 show the cells mounted in boxes, each case containing fifty cells, and that in Fig. 92 having also a small induction coil attached.

In the use of batteries it often becomes important to arrange a number of cells in such a way that through a given external resistance we may obtain the largest possible current. We have found from Ohm's law that the current which is furnished by a

Fig. 91.-cells Joined In "seiues." certain electro-motive force is not only dependent upon the electro-motive force itself, but also upon the resistance through which the current must flow. Hence, since the internal resistance of the battery must be included in the circuit, the maximum current is not a question of the heaping up of electro-motive forces, but of arranging the cells so that the electro-motive force is greatest when the resistance is least. Now, cells can be arranged in three ways: they can be joined with their poles positive to negative, positive to negative, and so on, in a chain, which is called arrangement "in series" (Fig. 95); they can be joined, all the positives and all the negatives together, called "in multiple arc" or "abreast" (Fig. 96), or, finally, they can be joined partly in series, partly abreast (Fig. 97).

Series Arrangement—Suppose we have « cells joined, as shown in the figure 95, *i.e.,* the copper of one coll to the zinc of the next, and so on. Let the electro-motive force of each

SERIES, MI'LTIPLE-ARC, COMBINATIONAL ARRANGEMENTS. 105 cell be E, its internal resistance r; and suppose the external resistance is R. Then we have evidently a battery with n times the electro-motive force and n times the internal resistance of a single cell. Hence, by Ohm's law the current is

$$\frac{nE}{R + nr}$$

Now, if R is small compared with r, the value of this does not differ greatly from "; that is, from ':; hence the current from n cells is, in this case, but a slight increase over the current from one cell, and no advantage has been gained by the process. But if R is very great compared with $n r$, then the fraction becomes nearly-, so that it is almost n times as great as if we had used only a single cell. Hence, in this case, *i.e*

, when the external resistance is great, there is an advantage in using a large number of cells in scries.

Multiple-Arc Arrangement—In this arrangement all the zinc poles *(Z)* are joined to one wire and all the copper poles (C) to another, these two wires themselves forming the new poles (Fig. 96). In this way the electro-motive force remains the same as before, i.e., that of a single cell, 2?, but the internal resistance, supposing there are n cells, has been diminished n times. The effect of joining the cells in this way is to make one large battery or cell, the area of whose plates has been increased »-fold. If the external resistance remains, as before, equal to R, we have again, bv Ohm's law, E

Current = and, as before, the current obtainable depends upon the relation of R to r,—*i.e.,* of the external to the internal resistance. Thus, if R is great compared with r, there is no advantage in joining the cells in this way. But if R is small compared with;, the current will by this means be increased nearly n times, exactly the reverse of what occurred with the arrangement in series.

Combinational Arrangement.—In this ease the cells are arranged partly in series and partly in parallel (Fig. 97). Suppose we have $n m$ cells in all, and of these m are joined in series, and therefore n in parallel. Then we have, by the application of Ohm's law to the case, supposing the external resistance to be Ii, and the internal resistance of one cell r, $R +. ,,-n R--m r$ and, as before, the value of the method of joining the cells depends entirely upon the relations existing between R and $/.$; that is, between the total resistance of the battery and the external resistance. When the latter is known, the best way to join up

Fig. 97.—Thkee Cells In "series," Two In "parallel." the battery is to make its final resistance as nearly as possible equal to the given external resistance. This equality can always be approximated to, and the more nearly equal the resistances may be, the larger will be the current from the battery through that particular external resistance.

This ride does not apply to the storage battery, because we have in this case to consider also the maximum discharge-rate for which the cells are suited. Their internal resistance is so low as to be generally negligible, and if the external resistance should have about the same value, the cells would be "short-circuited" and probably be irretrievably damaged.

CHAPTER IV.

Storage Electricity. *Storage Batteries, or Accumulators.*—We have a clear foreshadowing of the storage battery (Figs. 98, 99, 100) in the experiment mentioned on page 91, in which it was observed that a reversed current of electricity could be produced by two platinum plates immersed in dilute sulphuric acid after the primary current

FlOS. 98 And 99.—Stoeage Cells. has been stopped, and the plates subsequently joined by a metallic wire outside the fluid. In this case, the very marked enfeeblement of the primary current, as well as the production of the reverse current, was traced to the action of the layers of gas deposited on the surface of the plates. It was pointed out, however, that there was probably no chemical combination between the gas and the plates, though this condition was approached in the close relation existing between the film and the plate.

This state of things differs from the phenomena occurring in the storage battery, inasmuch as in the latter there *is* a chemical change going on at the surface of the two plates which affects the plates themselves; and it is upon this change—as long as it is a reversible one—that the value of the battery depends.

It is, therefore, altogether erroneous to call an apparatus, made as the so-called storage battery is made, a storage battery or accumulator, or to speak of stored electricity at all under these circumstances. There occurs, as far as we know, no storage of electricity whatever in this or in similar cases; indeed no electrification can be observed in the plates of which the battery is composed. In other words, the "storage" cell has become the seat of a more or less reversible *chemical change,* and as long as chemical action is prevented there is no electricity in the cell.

The only known apparatus, as far as electrical devices are concerned, which may be properly called a storage battery, is the Leyden jar. Here, as well as in similar arrangements called condensers, there is an actual accumulation of electricity, and the quantity which can be thus "accumulated" or "stored up," upon a given area, depends upon the distance apart of the surfaces and the nature of the medium between them, but not on the nature of the conductor itself.

Nothing of this kind holds true in the storage battery, but, as the apparatus referred to by that name is so well known, it will be advisable to retain the term.

Plante Type of Cell.—Some years ago a French electrician, Gaston Plante, constructed a storage cell which may be said to have been the first practical one (Fig. 101). This was made of two sheets of lead immersed in dilute sulphuric acid. Through this arrangement an electric current was passed for a certain length of time, alter which it was found that one plate had become oxidized, the other remaining practically unaffected. Then the current was passed through the cell in the opposite direction, with the result of oxidizing the plate before unacted upon, and of reducing the oxide previously formed on the other plate to the condition of spongy lead. The process was repeated a number of times, and it was found that the capacity of the cell—that is, the length of time it would furnish a current of a given intensity—was increased, within certain limits, proportionately to the number of times the charging operations were repeated. The final result of the action of the charging current was seen to be the formation of a rather thick layer of spongy lead on one plate, and of lead oxide on the other. Two plates in this condition are ready for use in the storage battery of the Plante type. The plates are then said to be "formed," and the operation just described is known as the process of "forming the plates." The plate with the layer of oxide upon it is called the *positive plate,* and that with the spongy lead the negative plate; that is to say, during discharge the current flows *from* the plate containing the oxide, through the circuit, and *into* the cell again by means of the spongy-lead plate. But during the process of charging the current flows *into* the cell through the positive plate, i.e., the oxidized plate, and *out* through the other. Now, during the charging operation, the positive plate becomes partly oxidized, the negative being more or less reduced to the condition of spongy lead. During the ensuing discharge the positive plate has a portion of its oxide reduced to a lower form of oxide, and some of it is reduced to spongy lead, while the negative plate is partially oxidized.. Thus, there is an alternate change, backward and forward, from lead to oxide of lead, and from oxide of lead to metallic lead again, which, as before remarked, is the essential feature of the storage battery.

Faure's Cell.—The Plante battery has the objection of requiring a very long time for the process of formation. To avoid this, Faure, also a French electrician, conceived the idea of coating the plates mechanically with lead salts, so that he could by this means materially shorten the time subsequently required to bring the plates into the proper condition.

At first Faure simply coated the lead sheets with lead oxides, so that there was but little mechanical support for these salts. Later, he employed plates with holes cut into them, technically called "grids," and plates of this kind, variously modified, especially in regard to the shape of the cavities, are at present almost exclusively employed.

In the cell as now used the lead plates are cast into molds of the required shape, their size varying with the kind of cell. After the plates are cast they are filled in with the lead oxide, or "active material," as it is called. This consists simply of an oxide of lead mixed with sufficient sulphuric acid to render it somewhat pasty. The paste is then mechanically pressed into the cavities of the plate, which are then rendered smooth. Two oxides of lead are generally employed: for the plate, which is to become, in the cell, the positive electrode, red lead Pb_3O_i is used; while in the negative plate there is used the yellow oxide, PbO. After these oxides have been suitably "filled" into the plates, the latter are regularly "formed" by passing a current of given intensity through them when immersed in dilute sulphuric acid. On the completion of this process the plates are ready for use.

Sometimes, in the manufacture of storage-battery plates, the interstices, instead of being cast into the plates, are the result of mixing some compound soluble in water with the molten lead (such as common salt, NaCl) and afterward dissolving this out. In this way the resulting pores are of irregular form, and appear capable of retaining the oxides of lead, afterward pressed in, more effectually than the pores of the usually regular shape. The plates of the storage cell arc all connected in parallel; that is, the positive plates are all joined by a lead strip, forming one electrode, the negative plates being joined in a similar way to another strip, so as to make up the other electrode. Any number of plates can, of course, be joined together, with the result of increasing the area of the electrodes a proportionate number of times, and this increase means a corresponding diminution in the internal resistance of the cell itself.

The chemical reactions which go on in the storage battery are still incompletely known, but it seems generally believed by those who have given the subject the most careful.study that the chemical changes do not end with the conversion of Pb_3O_4 into-PbO_2 on the positive plate, and of PbO into Pb on the negative. There is always a quantity of sulphate of lead formed, during discharge, on both plates, and, according to Gladstone and Tribe, and others, this reaction is that on which the working of the battery depends. It has been found that, after discharge has been continued to a certain extent, there is on the negative plate a mixture of spongy lead and sulphate of lead, and on the positive a mixture of sulphate and undecomposed lead oxide. These changes may be represented by the chemical equation, $Pb + 2Ha80t + Pb0a = 2PbS0t + 2Ha0$

In support of this view, it can be readily proved that the dilute acid in which the plates are immersed always grows weaker during the discharge of the cells.

While the cells are charging the reverse phenomena occur, namely, on the positive plate the sulphate becomes oxidized with the formation of sulphuric acid, thus: $PbSOt + 0 + ZT2O = PbO_2 + HuSOi$ and on the negative the sulphate hecomes reduced also with the production of sulphuric acid, $PbSOt + 7/2 = Pb + H2SOt$

There is, further, a local action going on at the surface of the plates, between the metal of the "grid" and the lead oxide on the positive electrode itself, $Pb + PbO2 + 2H2SOt = 2PbSOt + 2F2O$

Here, also, there is a formation of sulphate of lead. This phenomenon offers an explanation of the well-known fact that in a storage cell the "formation " of the plates frequently continues even after the current has been stopped.

Another important reaction taking place in these cells is the formation, of peroxide of lead on the negative plate, which results from the oxidation of sulphate during discharge. It is this formation which causes the phenomenon of residual discharge, so marked in most forms of storage cell. The peroxide of the negative plate tends to establish equilibrium between itself and the positive plate, even before the sulphating is complete and before the positive peroxide has disappeared. Thus the electromotive force gradually falls. But after an interval of rest the negative peroxide becomes converted into sulphate, from the local action between itself and the metallic lead, and the electro-motive force reaches its normal value again. Thus the cell is once more able to furnish a large current, with, however, a recurrence of the same series of phenomena.

This action increases with increase in the discharge-rate; hence, the electromotive force falls very rapidly when very heavy currents are taken from the cell.

The electro-motive force of the lead, lead-oxide storage cell, varies considerably with the conditions under which the cell is used. In ordinary working the electro-motive force may be taken as equal to 2 volts.

During charge, especially toward the end of the process, the electro-motive force rises much above this value, and when the cell is discharging it falls below, and continues to do so until, when completely discharged, its electro-motive force is zero. The figure (102) represents two curves taken at random from a series of tests of several well-known types of storage batteries. The curve A shows how the electro-motive force rises *during charge* until it reaches the value of about 21-volts, after which a further continuation of the process is a waste of current. Curve B represents the variation of electro-motive force during a discharge. It will be seen that, according to this, the potential remains rather constant at about 1.90 or 1.95 volts for the greater part of the time of discharge, and that when it begins to fall it falls very rapidly. These discharge curves are, however, very indeterminate, since their form depends altogether upon the intensity of the current taken from the battery. If this is great the electro-motive force falls very rapidly, and even at the start diminishes perceptibly in short intervals of time. On the other hand, if it is small, the electromotive force remains nearly constant at approximately 2 volts for nearly the whole time of discharge.

In the practical use of the battery it is advisable never to push the discharge so far as indicated on this curve. When the electro-motive force falls to 1.8 or 1.7 volts the battery should be disconnected and *at once* recharged, for the battery sutlers when, in disuse, it is in an uncharged state.

The capacity of a storage battery is generally measured in ampere-hours; that is, by the number of hours it will supply a current of given intensity. Thus, a battery whose capacity is said to bo 100 ampere-hours is one which will furnish a current of 10 amperes for 10 hours, or a current of 5 amperes for 20 hours, or a current of 25 amperes for 4 hours. These examples are, however, not all identical, for a cell which might give 10 amperes for 10 hours, would probably give 25 amperes for only 3 hours, and 50 amperes, perhaps, during only 1 hour. In other words, the capacity diminishes with the intensity of the current used, just as the electro-motive force was shown to do. Moreover, it is usual on the part of the manufacturers to specify the intensity of the current which they believe best suited for their cells, and the capacity of the battery reaches its normal value only when the discharging current does not exceed this.

The value of the current which the cell is best suited to furnish depends upon the character of the plates and their size and number, and is called the discharge-rate. A higher rate can be used for discharging than for charging without detriment to the cell. It is determined, as stated, for a particular cell by the size and number of the plates, and is based upon a current of given intensity per square centimetre of surface of plate. It has been found that when this value of the current is exceeded there is much waste of energy in the decomposition of the water and other irreversible actions, as well as a rapid deterioration of the plates.

The discharging rate best adapted to the ordinary lead plate (pasted), as now made, is about 25 amperes per seven square feet of total surface.

When a current of this proportionate value is employed the cells do no "boil" perceptibly—that is, do not freely give off gas, which of course represents a dissipation of part of the energy of the current—until the charging is complete. The cell is completely charged when its electro-motive force—with proper charging rate—reaches the value of 2.5 volts; after this, whatever current is put into the cell is wasted.

On the other hand, if a too weak current is used, there is again much waste of energy, and. indeed, the charge, as measured in ampere-hours, may greatly exceed that which the cell ought to obtaiu.

This is due to defective insulation, which it is almost impossible to completely guard against; however, as a chargingrate which is too small means simply a loss of energy, while an excessive rate means, in addition to this, great danger to the life of the battery, we should be, on the whole, carefid to liave the error on this side.

The internal resistance of the ordinary form of commercial storage battery is very low, being, for a cell with 19 plates of the size 7 by 9 inches, about. 002 or.003 of an ohm. It varies with the number of plates, *i.e.,* the total surface exposed to the current, and with their distance apart, and is a little greater during charge than discharge. It is, therefore, impossible to state its value accurately unless these conditions are known.

As stated, the density of the acid surrounding the plates becomes greater and greater as the charging progresses, and when the cell is fully charged it should reach the value 1200 Baume.

In replenishing the liquid it is only necessary to add water to the cell, unless by excessive " bubbling " some acid may have been thrown out. In general, only the water is lost, since the acid does not evaporate, and hence we have only to replace this. The average density of the solution should be about 1175, and when it falls to near 1100 the cell should be immediately recharged.

For some classes of medical work, and in such other work as may require currents ranging from '25 milliamperes up to 2000 or 3000, a storage-cell, similar to that shown in Fig. 103, is very suitable. These cells contain three or five plates,—two or three negatives and one or two positives,—and are provided with a screw or India-rubber cap at the top, through which the gases formed during charge can escape. The case itself is of "hard rubber," and is almost water-tight, the only opening being the cap, which is removed only when necessary. The dimensions of these cells are about as follow: Fig Im Height, seven inches; width, four inches; thickness, three inches; and each cell weighs about ten or fifteen pounds. The capacity is about two or three ampere-hours, so that even at the maximum rate for which these small cells are intended they will furnish a current of 1 ampere continuously for at least two or three hours. As in all storage batteries, so in this type, the electro-motive force for an average discharge is about two volts. When these cells are employed regularly it is advisable to have two batteries of the required number of cells, so that one battery may be charged while the other is in service. If it is necessary to employ an electro-motive force of 80 or 100 volts, forty or fifty of these cells could be arranged in a case of not excessive size. These cells are also very useful when it is desired to use a search-lamp (Fig. 104) for illuminating the cavities of the human body. One electric lamp furnishing a light equal to about one candle can be easily supplied from two of these cells, and kept burning continuously for about three hours. The lamps must be mounted on a suitable frame, which should have a key by means of which the current could be turned on or off, as desired.

Electrical Units.—It has been shown on page 6 that, provided all the quantities are measured in the same units, we can write, for the force acting between two bodies whose charges are q and qY and whose distance apart is r, *ra*

We must therefore define our unit of force. This is done according to Newton's first law of motion, which is stated thus: The unit force is that force which, acting for unit time on the unit mass, produces unit velocity. It therefore depends upon the units of length, of mass, and of time. At the present day these are, throughout the entire scientific world, the centimetre for unit length, the gramme for unit mass, and the second for unit time. The first two are included in the French system of measurement. In terms of these units, therefore, Newton's law may otherwise be stilted in these words: The unit force is that force which, acting for one second on a mass of one gramme, produces a velocity of one centimetre per second. This is called one Dyne, and the system of measurement based on these units is called the absolute system.

Hence, we define the unit quantity of electricity as that quantity which will exert on an equal quantity, placed one centimetre from it, the force of one dyne.

The unit potential is, therefore, the potential at a point one centimetre away from a unit charge, since r On a very small body.

These electrical units, being based upon the unit quantity of electricity and the force exerted by two units at a unit distance apart, arc called electro-static units. We can, however, base our measurements upon the unit magnetic pole, defining the unit pole in the same way, by calling it that pole which exerts on another similar pole at unit distance the unit force.. This system of units is called the electro-magnetic system. Xow, it is found in practice that the unit current, and the unit electro-motive force, and the unit resistance, when founded on the so-called absolute units, or, better, the C., G., S: (meaning centimetre, gramme, second) system, are either too small or too large for ordinary use. Electricians have, therefore, adopted certain multiples or submultiples of these as being more convenient for the purposes of electrical measurement; and we must not think on this account that there are too many standards, nor that those which have been selected finally are unnecessarily arbitrary. The value of any system of units is dependent upon the extent to which it is accepted throughout the world, and by this ride the value of the absolute system is great indeed, since it is the only system used to express *scientific* measurements. The so-called practical units adopted by electricians everywhere, and based on the C., G., S. system, are now universally" employed in the measurement of electrical quantities. Therefore, a current or a resistance, when measured at any place, is directly comparable with any other current or resistance measured at some widely different place.

As stated, in the electro-magnetic system of units the quantities, current, resistance, potential, etc., are deducible from the laws of the action of two magnetic poles upon each other, and of the action of a current of electricity on a magnetic needle suspended near it.

From these two laws, and the application of Ohm's law, given on page 32, we can at once define the units referred to. Those which are actually used in practice are, however, given in the following table, together with their relations to the C., G., S. units:—
ELEC'TUO-MAGNETIC SYSTEM.
Name of Unit. Equivalent in C, G., S. Units.

Resistance (Ohm),.... 1,000,000,000 = 10s

Current (Ampere),... iV == 1_1
Electro-motive foree (Volt),.. 100,000,000 = 10"8
Quantity (Coulomb),... a = 10_I
Capacity (Farad),... To-buowbs =,0-3

These practical units are again subdivided for convenience, and new values are used, whose relation to these is found by multiplying or by dividing the particular unit by one million. When it is multiplied the term mega is prefixed to the unit to express this fact, and when divided the term micro is used. Thus, one mega-ohm, or megohm, as it is written, means 1,000,000 ohms, and is a quantity very much used in the measurement of high resistances, such as the insulation resistance of wires and cables covered with India-rubber or gutta-percha compounds, etc.; that is to say, the word megohm is used to express the resistance of comparative non-conductors. As a rule, however, we have to deal with resistances much less than a megohm, so that they can usually be expressed as so many ohms. According to the most recent determination of this unit, an ohm is the resistance of a column of pure mercury one square millimetre in cross-section and 106.25 centimetres long, at a temperature of 10 C. Some practical idea of the value of an ohm may be formed, from the statement that the resistance of a pure copper wire 485 metres long and 1 millimetre in diameter is almost exactly an ohm.

The unit of electro-motive force, the volt, is seldom used as a multiple or a submultiple. The electro-motive force of a Daniell cell in good order, or of a chloride of silver element, is almost exactly one volt, and that of a storage cell while discharging is about twice this.

The ampere, the practical unit of current, is also seldom subdivided, except, however, in medical electricity, where the one-thousandth of an ampere, called a milliampere, is the unit generally adopted. For most medical work an ampere would be an excessive current, except in the employment of the cautery, and for convenience physicians prefer to give the results of their measurements in terms of milliamperes, and, sometimes, centiamperes.

Instead of the term "farad," the unit of capacity, the onemillionth of a farad, called a microfarad, is generally employed, as this corresponds more nearly with the capacity of those condensers, cables, etc., which are in practical use. Thus, the capacity of most submarine cables is about one-third microfarad per knot.

The coulomb is the unit quantity of electricity, and is used in voltameter measurements, and electrolytic work in general, where we have to express the *quantify* of electricity which has decomposed a given weight of substance. When a current of one ampere flows for one second of time, the *quantity* of electricity which has passed through any cross-section of the circuit is one coulomb. And, in general, the quantity of electricity which has passed, expressed in coulombs, is found by multiplying the current expressed in amperes by the time in seconds during which the current has continued to flow-.

The quantities, ampere, volt, ohm, are all deducible, any one when two others are given, by the application of Ohm's law. Thus, if in a circuit whose resistance is 1 ohm we have acting an electro-motive force of one volt, the current will be _ one volt $V = $ —7— = one ampere,
one ohm l

Or, if the resistance were 14.000 ohms, and the electromotive force 5G volts, then the current would be given by the equation 50 volts 4 $C = $ TTTi»in" i — = rsvm =-004 amperes,
14,000 ohms 1000 '
which we could also write 4 milliamperes.

Again, if by one galvanometer, or, as

it is sometimes called, milliamperemeter, or, still more shortly, mil-ammeter, we find the current to be 23 milliamperes, and also know that the electro-motive force of the battery is, say, 40 volts; then by Ohm's law we can find the resistance of the entire circuit at once from the equation $R = J$; hence, $R = 40\text{-f- (j}$, and not simply 23, because the current is expressed in milliamperes, and not in amperes, as it should be to correspond with volts and ohms). Carrying this out, we have $-1 = 1739$ ohms, nearly, which is, therefore, the resistance of the entire circuit.

Finally, if the current was found to be 3 milliamperes, and the resistance determined to be 24,000 ohms, we find for the electro-motive force acting in circuit, by the equation (Ohm's law) $E = CR$: $E = X\ 24{,}000 = 72$ volts (writing for the same reason as explained above).

The unit of work or energy is called the ""Watt," and is expressible in mechanical units; that is, in terms of one horsepower, by the relation: 746 watts = 1 horse-power, or 1 watt = Tg horse-power.

Now, as we know, electrical energy is measured by the product of current and electro-motive force, the units of which are, respectively, the ampere and the volt. Hence, a current of one ampere flowing under a difference of potential of one volt is giving out energy at the rate of 1 watt. If the current had been 10 amperes, and the electro-motive force in any part of the circuit had been, say, 60 volts, the rate of expenditure of energy would have been $60\ XK' = 600$ watts, which is equivalent to $Yij = .804$ horse-power, or approximately of one horse-power. This is about the rate of consumption of power in the ordinary electric light (arc-lamp) used in the streets of our cities. The incandescent lamp of about sixteencandle-power requires something like one-half to three-quarters of an ampere, and usually an electro-motive force of 110 volts. In practice from ten to fourteen of these lamps are regarded as equivalent to one horse-power.

Thermo-Electricity.—It has long been known that two metals, when joined so as to form a complete circuit, the two junctions being at different temperatures, have an electro-motive force set up at one of the junctions, so that an electric current flows in the circuit. Thus, in Fig. 105, if A represents a bent rod of one metal and B a similar rod of another metal, and if either junction JJ or Jt is heated, the other being kept cool, a current will flow in the circuit so made up, and its direction will be determined by the nature of the metals and their mean temperature. Two metals, arranged as in the figure, constitute what is known as a thermo-electric cell. Currents produced in this way are called thermo-electric currents, and the electro-motive force upon which such currents depend is itself, as just stated, dependent upon the nature of the metals employed, upon the mean temperature of the two metals, and upon the difference in the temperature of their junctions.

According to the direction in which the current flows across the hot junction of the different metals, the latter are divided into two groups. If, in Fig. 105, we suppose the current to flow from A to B across the junction J, this being the hot junction, then the metal A is said to be thermo-electrically positive to B. Or, we can state that B is thermo-electrically negative to A. That is to say, one metal is thermo-electrically positive to another if across the hot junction the direction of the current is from this one to the other. The two states are, however, merely relative, and a metal which is thermo-electrically positive to another given metal may, under different circumstances, become itself negative to the same metal.

We can, however, arrange a large number of metals in a series, which, for any mean temperature, will show their relation to each other, and in which each metal is thermo-electrically positive to those following in order.

In the construction of these tables it is usual to employ some metal as a standard of reference, and to determine in arbitrary units the values of the electro-motive force, or the thermoelectric power, as we may call it, of other metals, at some fixed temperature, to this one.

The following table is based upon Matthiessen's experiments, and the numbers express, approximately, the electro-motive force in microvolts (iinriTFinF volts) per degree centigrade of the different elements taken with respect to lead:—

MEAN TEMPERATURE, 20.
Bismuth (pressed),-(-97.
Cobalt, 22..
Lead, 0.
Tin, — 0.1
Commereial copper, — 0.1
Antimony (pressed), — 2.8
Silver (pure), — 3.
Antimony (crystals), — 24.5
Selenium, — 807.

These numbers are, however, by no means constant, but change with the mean temperature of the metals.

Thermo-electric currents have been practically applied so far only as a means of showing small differences of temperature, and for this purpose a thermo-electric cell is an extremely useful arrangement. It is at once evident that, instead of employing a single cell, composed of two metals (antimony and bismuth are the metals universally used), we could, as in the case of the galvanic battery, join up any number of such elements end to end, and form thus a thermo-electric battery (Fig. 106), where A, A, A are the antimony strips and B, B, B the bismuth. In this way we can add the electro-motive forces due to all the pairs and make it as great as we please. The metals are arranged as shown in the figure, a number of small rods of antimony and bismuth being joined with their bent ends, and several rows of these placed in a square frame, one over the other. The junctions at one side of the frame are exposed to the source of heat, and the two ends of the series of rods at the other side of the frame are fastened to copper wires leading to a galvanometer (Fig. 107). Under these circumstances, even when the source of heat is compara

Fig. 107.— Thermo-Electrical ApParatus (thermopile.) tively far removed,—so far, indeed, as to leave a sensitive thermometer entirely unaffected,—the galvanometer, if a proper one is used, will give an appreciable deflection and show $8L$ M clearly that the junctions have become warmed. These currents are generally small, but, by using thick and short rods of antimony and bismuth, and by employ ing many elements, currents of considerable magnitude can be obtained, because in this case the internal resistance of the thermo-electric battery would be considerably reduced.

Motors and Dynamos.—We have already given the general theory of the dynamo-electric machine (Figs. 108 and 109) on page 82, on which was explained the production of electromotive force by the movement of a conductor in a magnetic field. It was there shown that if we.move a wire near a majrnet, or move a magnet near a wire, an electro-motive force will be established between the ends of the wire, tending to urge a current along it. It was further shown that the direction of the electro-motive force acting depended upon the relative direction of the magnetic field, and that its value was dependent both upon the velocity of motion across the field and the strength of the field.

Upon these few and easily demonstrable facts the action of all dynamo machines and electric motors is based, and the complexity of some of them is brought about simply by the various demands of practice and the observance of details. We have, then, first to consider in every dynamo or motor the magnets *MM* (Fig. 110), which are either permanent or temporary, *i.e.,* electro-magnets, and, secondly, the armature, *A,* which consists of a coil of copper wire wound over a core of soft iron. The ends of the magnet between which the armature rotates are called its poles, *P* P(Fig. 110), and the aim is so to construct the magnets that the magnetic field in which the armature moves shall, under given conditions, be as strong as possible. C, *C, C, C* (Fig. 110) represent the coils of wire—"magnetizing coils "—around the magnet.

The armature consists of a number of soft-iron washers or disks (Fig. 112) covered with paper on one side and threaded on

Fig. 112.—Siemens' Armature. a steel rod, which forms the axle of the armature and moves in bearings at its ends. The washers, after being threaded on the rod, are pressed together and kept in place by means of two screws at the ends; occasionally they are *shrunk* on the shaft or axle. An armature of this kind is known as the Siemens' armature, and is, perhaps, the most generally used at present.

Another style of armature, called the Gramme ring (Fig. 113), is made of similar disks, or often wire, but with a larger opening in the centre, and the disks are afterward held to the axle by means of wedges, generally of wood.

In both cases this iron framework is wound with insulated wire,—in the Siemens' armature longitudinally, and in the Gramme form around the ring, part of the wire being thus inside and part outside, *i.e.,* external. Tins will be understood from the figure (113), in which is shown a Gramme armature cut through so as to make clear its structure.

In order to lead the current from the armature and to reverse its direction at the proper time the ends of the separate turns of wire are brought to a contrivance on the end of the axle called the commutator, marked *C* in Fig. 114. The commutator is made up of bars of copper like the spokes of a wheel, but not touching at any point, each bar or "segment," as it is called, being insulated from its two adjacent neighbors. At two diametrically opposite points on the commutator; and pressing against it, are metal strips technically called "brushes," *B B* (Fig. 114), which serve the purpose of leading the current to or from the armature (according as the machine is used as a motor or dynamo) as it revolves around.

Fig. 115.—Armature Revolving, Showing Lines Of Force.

As the armature consists of a mass of soft iron, around which circulates an electric current, we should expect it would become magnetized during passage of the current. This is really the case, and the current flows in such a direction that the poles of the armature are continually at right angles, or nearly at right angles, to the poles of the magnets themselves (Fig. 115). This is accomplished by the aid of the commutator, by means of which the direction of the current in the separate wires of the armature is When a particular wire of the armature passes the north pole of the magnet, it has an electro-motive force acting in one direction; when it passes the south pole the electro-motive force acts in the opposite direction. The commutator enables the electro-inotivc forces thus produced to act all in one direction, so that the current derivable from such a machine, instead of being first in one direction and then in the opposite, is always flowing the same way.

« changed every time the corresponding.segment of the commutator passes the brush. In this way the armature '"core" is magnetized, so that its poles point up and down,—say, the north pole being uppermost. Now, since the field-magnets have their poles pointing sideways, the north pole, let us suppose, being to the left, there is a continual tendency for the armature to revolve, owing to the mutual action of the poles on each other. This is the mode of action of the electric motor. In the case of the dynamo we have only to remember that, when the armature moves, its wires cut across the lines of force which go from one pole of the magnet to the other, and hence must have an electro-motive force established in them.

In the dynamo the armature is made to revolve by the expenditure *of mechanical work,* and in the motor the armature is made to revolve by the expenditure of *electrical work.*

In nearly all motors and dynamos used to-day the employment of permanent magnets has been abandoned, for the reason that the magnetism of such magnets cannot be very intense, and hence tlie machines not very powerful. Furthermore, all permanent magnets, as stated before, gradually lose their magnetism, and, though they become more stable after long-continued use, they can never be said to be constant.

When electro-magnets are employed to produce the magnetic fields of motors and dynamos, the magnetizing current is led off from the armature, where it is produced, in one of two ways. In one method the armature, the field-coils, and the external circuit (where the current is used) are all in one continuous circuit. They are, in fact, in series, and the dynamo is called a *series dynamo* (Fig. 116), where *VA* represents the armature, *V* the wire around the magnets, and *R* the external resistance. In the other method the external circuit and the field-coils are in multiple are, or in shunt relation, and the dynamo is then called a shunt dynamo (Fig. 117). In the first case (Fig. 116) the current flows out from the armature *(VA)*, through the field-coils *(V)*, through the external circuit *(R)*, back to the armature. In the second case (Fig. 117) the current flows out from the armature (*VA)*, part going then through the field-coils *(Vs)* and part through the external circuit (2?), afterward uniting and flowing back through the armature. Shunt motors and dynamos receive often the name *constant potential machines,* because, when they are properly made, such machines, used as dynamos, give at constant speed a constant electro-motive force, and when used as motors and supplied with current at constant potential,—as, for instance, when joined to a number of storage cells,—run at a constant speed, no matter what work they may be doing. It is scarcely necessary to point out that most forms of motive apparatus tend to ran slower when doing heavy work than when doing light work, and very often such irregularity in speed is exceedingly objectionable. The extent to which this is overcome in electric motors is shown by the fact that many shunt motors, in general use, are so well constructed that their change in speed between full load and no load at all amounts to only a few per cent.

The armature axle is provided at one end with a pulley, which, by means of a belt or other suitable coupling, transmits the power to or from the armature, accoding as the machine is tised as a dynamo or as a motor. The pulley of the motor must be chosen of such a size, relatively to that of the apparatus to be driven, that the speed of the latter shall be what is desired. Many motors are fitted with controlling devices and regulating attachments, so that the speed may be varied at will between limits of a considerable range. This is sometimes a very essential feature.

The capacity of motors and dynamos is rated in horse-power units, and machines are now made by various manufacturing companies whose capacity varies from less than- of a horsepower to 100 or more horse-power.. It is thus possible to select a motor of such a size that it can be used for almost any variety of mechanical work.

The question of supplying motors with current is a very important one, and the subject has, within the last few years, received much attention. Many attempts have been made to employ primary batteries for the work, but so far with very doubtful success, even under the most favorable conditions. If batteries have to be used, there can be no doubt of the great superiority of the storage battery. The only serious objection which can be raised to these is their weight, which amounts to approximately six hundred pounds per horse-power. Portable storage batteries are, however, now manufactured which are capable of driving small motors, and which have been found quite satisfactory.

In some cases the electric-light current is available, either from a central station or from some neighboring plant, and under these circumstances motors may be supplied with current without any difficulty. It is altogether immaterial what particular system of electric distribution may be adopted at the station, since motors may be constructed in such a way that they can be joined to any circuit whatever. But, it must be added, the motor will have to be built in accordance with the conditions under which it will be supplied with current.

Resistance Coils, Rheostats, etc.—Resistance coils, sometimes called rheostats, rheotomes, etc., are made in great variety of form, according to the special purposes for which they are intended, but they are nearly always constructed so that the resistance in circuit may be varied at will between certain limits.

In some forms this can be done by a continuous variation, but usually the resistance must be changed by steps; that is, the resistance must be changed one or more ohms at a time. A resistance box of the latter kind is that shown in Fig. 118. It consists of a rectangular box with a hard-rubber top, having inside a number of spools of German-silver wire connected through the top with brass pieces of appropriate shape. The brass pieces *(A A)* are of the form shown in Fig. 119; they are placed close together, and contact from one to the other is made by inserting plugs (/?) into half-rounded cavities between them. The coils of wire forming the various resistances are joined one end to one block, and the other end to the next adjacent block, thus bridging across from one block to the other. In winding the coils it is usual to double the wire—which is always covered with some good insulating material—so that it is wound back on itself. That is to say, half the reel or spool is wound in one direction, and half in the opposite, the object of this being to reduce the self-induction (page 87) as much as possible. The nurrfber of coils of wire, as well as the value of their resistance, is generally such that any resistance from one ohm to one thousand or more can be thrown in circuit. Some boxes have coils with resistances from one to ten thousand ohms. In using these boxes the circuit wires are joined to the binding-posts with which the resistance boxes are provided, and the resistance is varied by removing or inserting plugs between the various blocks. When any plug is removed the current must flow through the particular resistance between the two blocks to which the plug belongs, and when the plug is inserted the resistance is practically out of circuit, so that the current flows directly across from block to block. In most of these boxes two of the blocks have no wire resistance between them; hence, when the plug between these two is removed, the resistance becomes infinitely great, and the current stops. This interval is marked *inf.* (= infinity).

A very similar form of resistance box is that indicated in Fig. 120. Here, instead of having plugs to remove and insert, there is a movable, metallic lever, which makes contact with a number of buttons between which are joined resistance coils of any desired value. The terminals to which the circuit wires are attached are marked 7j and T2. Of these, 7i leads directly to the last button of the series of resistances, and T2 to the axis of the lever. By moving the lever in one direction or the other we can make the current flow through as many of the resistances, ru ? etc., as we please, and break the current entirely by moving the lever to a position between any of the buttons. If the lever is allowed to rest on the button Bg all the resistances arc thrown out of circuit, and the current flows from T2 say, to A, through the lever-arm to Bn to 7J directly.

A resistance apparatus in which the changes are continuous is that known as the water-rheostat (Figs. 121 and 122), the principle of which depends upon a change in the sectional area of a liquid through which the current flows. Two metallic plates (Fig. 123), A and B, are immersed in water and joined by a wire; another plate, C, is capable of moving up and down between the plates A and B. To the latter is joined one circuit wire, and to the two plates A and B the other circuit wire. When the plate C is pushed downward as far as it will allow, the surface of water through which the current passes is as great as possible, the resistance has its minimum value, and the current its maximum. As C is moved upward the resistance continually increases, since the area becomes less and less, until finally, when it is moved above the level of the water, the current ceases altogether. The objection to rheostats of this kind is the polarization, which is sometimes excessive.

Switches.—It is often necessary, when experimenting with the electric current, to be able to make and break the circuit rapidly and whenever desired. To do this it is usual to insert into that part of the circuit which has to be thus changed an apparatus called a switch or contact-key. In its simplest form this is only a spring, S (Fig. 124), furnished with a knob, B, 1 one end of the spring: being: Fig. 124. ro o permanently connected with the circuit wire, D, the other making contact, and thus completing the circuit only when pressed down on the terminal of the wire, C The spring is fastened to a board as a base, and the two circuit wires pass through holes in this, to the top. In the position shown, the current cannot flow because the circuit is broken between the spring and the point, D. These keys are often provided with another spring-catch which keeps the main spring in contact with H, until it is desired to release it.

In order to be able to reverse the direction of the current without changing the connection of the wire with the battery or other source of electricity, there is inserted in the circuit what is known as a "reversing key," or " commutator" (Fig. 125), inu which by moving a hinged arm we can change the direction of the current at pleasure. The general principle of a key of this kind is shown diagramatically in the figure. Here, the main wires are joined to the points A and B. These points can be connected to the points F, G, ll, Khy the metallic arms C'and I), which are rigidly joined by an insulating connecting piece provided with a knob, E. The points F, G, H, K are joined by wires, as shown, with two other points, the latter, L and M, being places of attachment for the circuit wires. L is connected with F and A' and M is joined to G and //. When the pieces C and D are pushed to the left the current flows *out* from L through the circuit and *in* through M. When the lever is pushed to the right the current flows *out* from M through the circuit and *in* through L; that is, the direction of the current is reversed. Generally these reversing keys are constructed as exhibited in Fig. 126. The connections are as shown, and the only difference between this and the one in Fig. 125 is in the use of three points, E, F, G, instead of four; the points E and G being connected together by a wire. The contact levers are, however, as before, moved to the right or to the left, according as the current is to be sent in one direction or the other.

When two wires cross each othpr. without touching, the drawing is usually made in this way: -, and the wire having the loop is supposed to be above the other.

A very useful form of reversing key is that known as the "rocking commutator" (Fig. 127). This consists of a rectangular frame of insulating material, having six cavities hollowed out along its edges, these cavities (metallic cups are often employed) being filled with mercury. To the two centre cups are attached the battery wires, and to the end cups, as shown, the wires of the circuit. Into the cups are fitted two pieces of wire on each side, one being bent into a half circle, F, and joined at its centre with a straight piece, E. The wires are connected by an insulating rod, D. The wires can be pushed from one side to the other, and thus caused to "rock" on the centre piece, E. In this way the centre piece always remains in its own mercury cup, but the end pieces alternately make and break contact witli their cups when the " rocker," as we may term it, is moved from one side to the other. The mercury cups are connected together crosswise, as shown, Kx with K1H and K3 with Kt By moving the rocker from one side to the other, the current in the circuit, L, 3f, is reversed. In the position shown in Fig. 127, the current flows as follows: In Cto K,z to K3 to Kt out M; in at L to Kx to A to Kh out at (72 to the battery. If the key were pushed over on the other side the direction would he as follows: In at C to K to Ku out at L; in at M to K± to 7v5, *out* at (7l, to battery.

Still another form of reversing key is shown in Fig 129. This is known as the " double-plug key." In this key there are four brass quadrants fastened close together (but not touching) on a hard-rubber or other insulating block. Each quadrant is provided with a binding-screw, b (Fig. 128), to which the circuit wires are attached, and with two circular grooves on its sides.

'The grooves are opposite each other and form in pairs, orifices, into which can be fitted the keys or plugs, K. The plugs have a handle of hard rubber, and when in place make contact between the quadrants. The wires of the circuit are joined to the quadrants diagonally, and the direction of the current is reversed by moving the plugs from between one set of quadrants to the other; rather less conveniently than in some other forms of key. *Combinational Keys.*—It is often very convenient to have an arrangement by which it is possible, on moving a switch, to send through the circuit in use, either a continuous or an alternating current, *i.e.*, a " galvanic" or "faradic" current. A plan showing the contacts and wiring of such an arrangement is given in Fig. 130. Here *B* is the battery or source ot the galvanic current, *G* is the induction coil furnishing the faradic current, and A", and *IC2* are switches of the kind already described in Fig. 126. The numbers from 1 to 10 represent the metallic contacts or bindingposts to which the different wires are attached. To the screws 1 and 2 are attached the faradic-current wires, and to 9 and 10 are joined the battery wires, while the circuit wires are joined to *C* and *T).* The points are connected permanently by wires in the following way: 1 to 4 to 7; 2 to 3; 6 to 8 to 5; 9 to *B* and 10 to *A*. With the key *K* in the middle position the galvanic current is broken; if then *K2* is pushed to the left the faradic current flows through the main circuit. When *Kz* is pushed over to the right and *Kx* to either side the galvanic current is available, and is reversed by simply moving *Kx* from one side to the other.

Glow Lamps.—For purposes of illumination, in medical and surgical practice, there are many advantages afforded by the electric lamp. In medical work and generally, when there is needed a light of something like one or two candle-power, small electric lamps requiring an electro-motive force of about four volts and a current of perhaps one ampere arc found very useful. These lamps consist of a glass bulb (Fig. 131), exhausted very completely of air, containing within it a thin strip of carbon, which is attached by means of platinum wires, blown into the glass, with two electrodes. The electrodes are joined, when the lamp is in use, with the terminals of a sufficiently powerful battery, and the connecting wires are generally provided with a key of some kind so that the circuit can be opened or closed at pleasure. When the circuit is closed the current flows through the lamp connections, and in passing through the carbon filament heats it to such a degree as to raise it to a state of incandescence. Consumption of the carbon filament is rendered impossible by the great rarity of air, and hence of oxygen, in the glass bulb. These lamps, generally known as *"incandescent lamps"* are so manufactured that they can be used with any desired number of storage cells, from two upward. For surgical purposes, however, lamps requiring about two cells, *i.e.* , four volts, are perhaps the most suitable; they'are quite small and can be employed for illuminating the cavities of the human body. *Telephone.*—Quite recently instruments closely allied in their structure with the now well-known telephone have been introduced into medical practice. In order, however, to make clear their general plan and the electrical principles involved in their working, it will not be necessary to do more than describe ve.ry simply the main features of the ordinary telephone, in almost universal employment to-day. The action of the telephone depends upon the magnetic changes which take place in a piece of magnetized iron when a magnetic body—such as an iron plate—is caused to move or *s* vibrate near it. The vibration of the iron plate causes simultaneous disturbances of the magnetism of the magnetized body, and these disturbances have the effect of establishing electric currents in a coil of wire wound about the latter. The currents are led, by copper wires, to a perfectly similar arrangement in which the same changes, but in a reverse order, take place. Thus, in Fig. 132, let *A* represent an iron plate of circular form supposed fastened rigidly along its circumference. Let *B* represent an iron bar, wound over one end with a coil of wire, *C*. Now, suppose the bar is magnetized by the action of the coil, *C,* and let us suppose the plate, *A,* or a diaphragm, as it is generally called, to move either inward or outward. The result will be that the magnetism of the bar, *B,* will undergo a change; lines of force will cut across the wires of the coil, *C* (in one direction or the other according to the direction of movement of the diaphragm), and hence set up new electro-motive forces in the coil itself. Thus, the magnetizing current which we have supposed to circulate in the coil, *C,* will be increased or diminished, and if we now imagine these currents to be led around another bar of iron with a diaphragm in front of it, like the former, the diaphragm will be attracted or repelled by the bar and will thus vibrate in complete accordance with the vibrations of first plate. In the telephone the diaphragm is set in vibration by the voice; the sound-waves impinging against it set it into corresponding movement.

We have, then, these series of changes in the telephone: First, the vibrations of the air and diaphragm; second, magnetic changes; third, increase or diminution of a current; fourth, a variable current in the line or connecting wires, *L M;* fifth, magnetic changes again; sixth, vibrations of another diaphragm, and, finally, the production of sound-waves. In practice one apparatus is called the transmitter and the other the receiver, the transmitter being the apparatus spoken to and the receiver the one placed before the ear.

Microphone.—Closely, related to the telephone is the mechanisra known as the *microphone,* an apparatus which is used to increase the intensity of sound. Such a result is produced by the action of two points in a circuit through which a current is flowing, the electrical resistance between which is varied by the changing pressure existing between the points. The points are, in general, made of hard carbon, because then, small changes of pressure cause considerable changes of electrical resistance. In Fig. 133 is shown one form of microphone. *P* is a carbon pencil touching slightly two carbon blocks, *Cu C* above and below. The blocks have cavities hollowed out of them, into which the ends of the pencil project. The blocks are fastened to a frame, and the whole is firmly fixed to a base, *S,* which should be a regular sounding-board. Through the blocks and pencil a cur rent—furnished by a battery, *B*—is flowing, and in the circuit of this is included an ordinary telephonic receiver, *li.* The current, therefore, has to flow through the two points of contact between the blocks and pencil, and its intensity depends upon the resistance offered at these points. Now, the resistance itself depends upon the pressure between the points, so that finally the current-strength may be said to be dependent upon the pressure between the carbons.

When the sounding-board is agitated in any way it causes the carbon pencil to vibrate with it, thus producing changes in the pressure at the points, and therefore in the resistance. The current, in consequence, is subjected to corresponding fluctua tion, and acts on the receiver just as it would in an ordinary telephone, reproducing there the vibrations of the soundingboard.

Microphones have been made of extreme sensibility; a fly walking on the sounding-board can be very distinctly heard through the receiver in some instruments, and the ticking of a watch produces sounds of a disagreeable intensity.

Part II.

Electro-physiology, Electro-diagnosis,

AND

Electro-medical Apparatus.

CHAPTER I.

Electro-physiology. *Muscle Currents.*—If a strip of muscle be isolated from its connections and intercalated in a circuit containing a delicate galvanometer or other electrical measuring apparatus, a measurable quantity of electricity will pass which appears to have its source in the muscle; in other words, the muscle seems to be an electric generator or battery.

It has been found that this current will pass only when contact is made with the muscle at certain points. If a cylindrical muscle, the sartorius of a frog, for example, is taken and the tendinous ends cut off, it may be considered as having two poles and an imaginary line of division at a point equidistant from the two poles, and called the equator.

DuBois-Reymond and other physiologists to whom we are mostly indebted for our knowledge of these phenomena, regard them as inherent properties of living muscle. The fact that the electric organ of certain electric fishes, as the torpedo, electric eel, etc., appears to be simply modified muscular tissue, lends some probability to this view. There are reasons, however, for believing that the so-called muscle currents arc not present in the natural, uninjured state of living muscle, but are developed in consequence of some injury or modification of the vital condition of the muscle.

However interesting these phenomena may be to the physiologist, they have no bearing upon electro-therapeutics and need concern us no further in this place.

Electrotonus.—When a galvanic current is passed through a motor nerve it produces certain changes in the normal irritability and conductivity of the nerve, which are termed by lQ (145) physiologists electrotonus. The nerve so modified is said to be polarized, and the current is called a polarizing current. The phenomena of electrotonus may be briefly described as follows: The nerve through which a current is passing is in a state of increased irritability near the point to which the cathode is applied. This is technically termed catelectrotonus. In the vicinity of the anode the irritability is decreased, and this condition is termed anelectrotonus. This increase and decrease of irritability—or catelectrotonus and anelectrotonus—is more marked between the points of application of the electrodes than beyond this interpolar district.

Formerly much stress was laid upon the direction of the current, and physiologists as well as electro-therapeutists insisted strongly upon the varying effects of "ascending" and "descending" currents. At present, however, there is pretty general agreement that the direction in which the current passes— whether from periphery to centre (ascending), or from centre to periphery (descending)—is of little consequence. The varying effects observed are, it is generally believed, dependent altogether upon tjie electrode or pole used in making the test. In the normal condition of the nerve the cathode produces the more intense effect.

Some electro-therapeutists have endeavored to base a theory of the therapeutic action of electricity upon the observed phenomena of electrotonus, but these endeavors have not up to the present time been very successful. The results of experiments upon the nerve-muscle preparation of the frog do not seem to be in entire agreement with the effects of the electric current as observed in the healthy or diseased nerve of man. Hence it will be wise for the present to only take account of the results obtained by experiments and observations upon human beings, and not try to twist the facts of experimental physiology into the support of a therapeutic theory.

The nature of the change in the nerve which causes the electrotonic condition is not understood, but there are good reasons for believing that it is due to an electrolytic re-arrangement of molecules which modifies the power of transmission of impulses. If a sufficiently strong current is used the irritability of the nerve is entirely abolished, and impulses can neither be originated in nor transmitted through the electrotonized district.

Sensory, like motor, nerves are subject to the laws of electrotonus.

Effects of Electric Currents upon Nerves and Muscles.—Electrical stimulation of a motor nerve causes contraction of the muscles to which the nerve is distributed. When the current is sent through a sensory nerve pain is produced in the area of distribution of the nerve, and when a mixed nerve is the object of experiment both of these effects are produced. Stimulation of the sympathetic causes variations in diameter of the bloodvessels and contraction of other unstriped muscles. *Stimulation of Motor Nerves—Pfluger's "Law of*

Contraction." —If the cathode of a galvanic battery furnishing a current of moderate strength is applied over a nerve superficially located and easily accessible, *e.g.,* the ulnar nerve at the elbow, and the anode placed at an indifferent point,—the sternum is usually selected,—a contraction of the muscles supplied by the nerve stimulated will follow on closing the circuit. It is immaterial for the production of this effect whether the circuit be closed with the cathode, the anode, or in the metallic part of the circuit. If electrodes of definite size be used, say, a flat anode of thirty square centimetres area, and a cathode often square centimetres, the contraction of the muscles on closing the circuit is usually produced when a current of 2.5 milliamperes is used. With this strength of current, opening the circuit with the cathode, or opening and closing with the anode, will produce no contraction. If, now, the current be increased to 3.4 milliamperes the contraction will be produced on closing the circuit with the anode, while the cathodic closing contraction will be increased. Still further increase of the current to 3.5 milliamperes will bring about contraction on opening the circuit with the anode, while a current of 8.2 milliamperes will be necessary to cause contraction on opening the circuit with the cathode. This strength of current will likewise produce a contraction of some duration, technically called "tetanus," on cathodic closing. The anodic closing and anodic opening contractions do not always follow in regular succession,—sometimes one and sometimes the other appears first.

This more or less regular gradation of the effects of the current has been established by numerous experiments and has been formulated into a definite law which is of great importance to the electro-therapeutist, for by the variation in the electrical reaction of the nerves during disease the nature of the morbid condition is distinctly manifested to the observant physician.

Brenner, to whose acute reasoning and patient observation electro-therapy is so deeply indebted, constructed a formula of the law of electrical contraction, which is represented by symbols, as follows:—

Cathodic closing contraction (Ca. Cl. C.) 4.
Anodic closing contraction (An. Cl. C.) 2.
Anodic opening contraction (An. 0. C.) 2.
Cathodic opening contraction (Ca. 0. C.) 1.

That is to say, with the same strength of current the cathodic closing contraction would be four times the strength of the cathodic opening contraction; or, in other words, only one-fourth of the current required to produce a contraction on opening the circuit with the cathode would suffice to produce a closing contraction with the same pole. It will be seen that the anodic closing and anodic opening contractions are produced by the same strength of current, which is midway between that required to produce contraction on closing or opening the circuit with the cathode.

The symbols, inclosed in brackets, are generally used for the purpose of economy of space, and when once thoroughly fixed in the memory will readily stand for the words themselves.

The contraction produced by the galvanic current, unless the latter is of excessive strength, is quick and short,—almost momentary, in fact. This is an important fact to remember in a diagnostic point of view, as a modification in the character of the contraction is an unfailing sign of disease in the nerve.

In testing a nerve by the galvanic current the contractions produced are much stronger when the current is reversed with the commutator, without opening the circuit, than when the circuit is first broken and then the poles reversed. This reversal of current with closed circuit is known to electro-therapeutists as the voltaic alternation, and is usually indicated by the symbol V. A. In many of the therapeutic applications of electricity the employment of voltaic alternation, or voltaic alternatives, is extremely important on account of the highly stimulating effects thus produced.

In striking contrast to the single, quick contraction or jerk produced by the galvanic current, the faradic current produces a tonic, prolonged contraction, which lasts during the entire time the current is passing. This is due to the fact that the contractions caused by the closing and opening and reversal of the circuit follow each other in the faradic machine so rapidly that the muscle cannot return to a state of rest in the interval between the contractions, and thus the latter apparently become continuous.

For convenience of reference, a table of symbols used in tbis work is given here:—

Ca. Cl. C, Cathodic closing contraction.
Ca. O. C, Cathodic opening contraction.
Ca. Cl. Te., Cathodic closing tetanus.
An. Cl. C, Anodic closing contract'on.
An. O. C, Anodic opening contraction.
An., Anode.
An. O. P., Anodic opening picture.
An. Cl. P., Anodic closing picture.
An. O. Od., Anodic opening odor.
An. Cl. Od., Anodic closing odor.
An. O. Sd., Anodic opening sound.
An. Cl. Sd., Anodic closing sound.
An. O. Sn., Anodic opening sensation.
An. Cl. Sn.. Anodic closing sensation.
An. Cl. Te., Anodic closing tetanus.
Dur., Duration (of current).
It I)., Reaction of degeneration.
E., or E.in.f., Electro-motive force.
C., Current.
R., Resistance.
G. S., Galvanization of the sympathetic.
B. G., Brain galvanization.
Ca., Cathode.
Ca. Dur., Cathodic duration.
C. D., Coil distance.
, Diminuendo.
, Crescendo.
Ca. Cl. Sn., Cathodic closing sensation.
Ca. O. Sn., Cathodic opening sensation.
Ca. Cl. Sd., Cathodic closing sound.
Ca. O. Sd., Cathodic opening sound.
Ca. Cl. P., Cathodic closing picture.
Ca. O. P., Cathodic opening picture.
Ca. Cl. Od., Cathodic closing odor.
Ca. O. Od., Cathodic opening odor.
Ma., Milliampere.

V. A., Voltaic alternatives.

Muscles can be directly stimulated to contraction by electric currents. This has been experimentally demonstrated in animals by paralyzing the nerves with curare and then subjecting' the muscles to the action of an electric current. The direct muscular contraction differs from the neuro-muscular contraction in being slower, and requiring a more prolonged action of the current. In the next chapter the causes of this difference of action will be more fully considered.

No elevation of temperature results in a muscle through which a galvanic current is passing unless contraction of the muscle is produced. Whether certain modifications of nutrition can be brought about by such non-contractile currents has not yet been definitely established. The assumption is justified, however, that even the mildest currents do produce some modification of nutrition.

When the current is sufficiently strong to produce contraction of the muscle, there is an increase of temperature which is proportional to the intensity of the contraction. This rise of temperature is not due to the passage of the current, nor to the increased hyperaemia, but solely to the greater metabolic activity going on in the muscle consequent upon its contraction. A paralyzed or unused muscle wastes in consequence of defective nutrition; hence, in cases of paralysis, where volitional contraction of the muscles is impossible, these must be stimulated artificially in order to prevent atrophy. For this purpose electricity is an admirable stimulant.

Sensory nerves can be stimulated to their specific reaction, *i.e.*, the production of pain, either by applying the electrode to the trunk or the peripheral terminations of the nerve. The sensation is experienced, however, only at the periphery, and not in the trunk. It is probable, therefore, that the sensation in a contracted muscle is due to stimulation of the sensory fibres distributed in the muscular substance, and not to any specific "electro-muscular sensibility." *Resistance.*—When a galvanic current is sent through organic tissues, such as a portion of the human body, it encounters resistance (see Part I, page 34), just as when a current passes through a wire or other metallic conductor. The resistance of organic tissue is, however, immensely greater than that of a metallic circuit. Different portions cf this organic conductor have different degrees of resistance, as will presently be shown more in detaU. It must also be borne in mind that organic tissue conducts the current largely, if not altogether, by virtue of the electrolytic decomposition going on in the track of the current. (See page 49.)

The course of the current in the body is determined, just as in other conductors, by the relative resistance offered by the different tissues. The largest current will naturally pass through that tissue which offers the least resistance. In general terms it may be said that the more succulent tissues are the best conductors.

The resistance of the epidermis is greater than that of any other tissue of the body. Recent determinations of this resistance (by Giirtner and Jolly) have shown that the resistance of the two layers of the epidermis in the percutaneous application of electricity is about three hundred times as great as that of all the intervening tissues. Hence, in estimating the resistance of the body to an electric current, the tissues under the skin need not be considered at all, as the obstruction they offer to the passage of the current is relatively unimportant.

When the current has passed through the body for a short time the resistance rapidly diminishes; in other words, the current passes through more easily, as may readily be shown by a milliamperemcter in the circuit. It is supposed by most writers that this diminution of resistance is due to increased hyperemia and succulence of the tissues permeated by the current, but there is reason to believe that the electrolytic arrangement of molecules in the track of the current has some influence in rendering the passage of the current easier.

At the other extremity of the scale of resistance offered by organic tissues are the brain, eyeballs, and spinal cord. Each of these transmit the current with the greatest readiness.

Density.—The density of the current varies very markedly in different portions of an organic conductor. At the points of entrance and exit the density is greatest, diminishing to the minimum at that portion of the interpolar area where the cross

FIG. 134.—Intended to show the distribution and density of current when electrodes of the game size are employed.

Fig. 13a— Shows the difference in density at the two poles when electrodes of different size are employed.

Fig. 13H.—.Shows the current density when the electrodes are applied near together and upon the same side of the body.

section of the conductor is greatest. This point may or mav not be midway between the two poles. It depends largely upon the relative sizes of the electrodes, their distance apart, and the nature of the tissues themselves. The entire question of interpolar resistance in organic tissues demands a thorough investigation in view of recent observations.

Erb has endeavored to show diagrammatically the varying density of the current. These diagrams, which are here reproduced (Figs. 13-1, 135, 136), fail, however, to show the modifying influence of different tissues upon the variations of density of the current.

OBJECTIVE AND SUBJECTIVE EFFECTS OF ELECTRIC CURRENTS UPON THE COMMON INTEGUMENT.

Both galvanic and faradic currents cause pain, burning or tingling, contraction of the cutaneous muscles, and hyperemia at the points of application of the electrodes. Increase in strength of the galvanic current, or increased duration of its passage, will result in inflammation, and produce the chemical effects known as electrolysis.

The degree of pain produced depends not only upon the strength of the current, but upon the shape, size, and material of the electrode, and the portion of the body to which it is applied. In practice, it is found that moistening the electrodes with a warm saline solution reduces the pain by facilitating the transmission of the current, *i.e.,* diminishing the resistance of the epidermis.

The greater degree of pain produced by dry electrodes is owing to the greater density of the current which enters the skin at the mouths of the cutaneous glands, sweat-pores, or hairfollicles. Moistening and softening the epidermis furnish a larger number of points of entrance for the current by subdividing it, and thus diminishing its density.

Therapeutists avail themselves of the powerful stimulating properties, both direct and reflex, of currents of great density by using the electric brush (a small bundle of fine wires) as an electrode. "When the object is to stimulate the skin directly, or to produce a reflex or derivative effect upon deeper or distant organs, the electric brush or small, dry electrodes are used and lightly applied to the surface. On the other hand, if irritation of the cutaneous and sensory nerves is to be avoided, the electrodes should be of large area, well moistened with a warm saline solution, and pressed firmly against the skin. Any one can convince himself of the different effects produced by alternately grasping firmly and holding loosely in the hands the electrodes of a faradic machine.

The pain of the galvanic current is burning in character and more intense at the cathode; that of the faradic current is rather in the nature of a prickling or tingling, sensation. By increasing the strength of the current the sensation can be increased to the point of becoming insupportable.

The motor phenomena produced by the electric current upon the skin consist in contractions of the cutaneous muscles, throwing the skin into irregular prominences,—the familiar "gooseskin." When the current is applied to the breast or scrotum, prominence of the nipple and retraction of the scrotum are produced. AYhen the galvanic current is used these contractions soon disappear, but they are more persistent under the faradic current.

Upon the blood-vessels of the skin the current first produces a contractile effect and afterward acts as a dilator. There is anuemia as a primary, and hyperaemia as a secondary, effect.

The objective effects of the constant current upon the skin are said, by Ziemssen, to appear in the following order: Pallor with cutis anserina, hyperaemia, papular projection of the hairfollicles, and, finally, confluence of the papules to form wheals. If the current is sufficiently strong the chemical effects of the electrolytic current become evident. The difference of chemical action at the two poles is very marked. The skin under the cathode soon becomes raised into a blister, which enlarges both in area and elevation. The reaction of the vesicular fluid is alkaline. Should the current be strengthened or much prolonged, a brownish slough forms.

At the anode the inflammatory reaction is less intense, and the serum obtained from the wheal formed at the point of contact of the electrode with the skin has an acid reaction. The metal surface of the electrode becomes oxidized and corroded.

These chemical effects are due to the electrolvtic action of the current *(q. v.).* They are produced in all organic tissues, —skin, muscle, nervous tissue, bone, etc.

No thermic effects are produced by the electrolytic current unless muscular contraction is produced. This has been experimentally demonstrated by Ziemssen, and is a result of daily experience in electro-therapeutics.

PHYSIOLOGICAL EFFECTS OF ELECTRIC CURRENTS UPON THE NERVES
OF SPECIAL SENSE.

Optic Nerve.—In testing the electrical reaction of the nerves of special sense the galvanic current is usually employed. The optical effects produced by the current differ with the electrode used. Most of the definite knowledge upon this subject we owe to the masterly researches of Brenner. With one electrode at the nape of the neck or to the sternum, and the other applied in the vicinity of the eye or over the closed lids, a sensation of colored light is produced in the eye tested. The sensation of color is subjective, and not objectively visible to the experimenter. With Ca. CI. the colors are a light-blue centre and a yellowish-green halo a little to the outer side of the visual axis. Reversal of the current produced a reversal of the relations of the colors; thus, on An. CI., the centre is yellowish green and the halo light blue. An. O. produces the same color-reaction as Ca. CI., and An. CI. the same as Ca. O. Every electrician is familiar, also, with the momentary flash of light caused by closing or opening a circuit through or in the vicinity of the eyeball. *Auditory Nerve.*—A sound sensation is caused by the galvanic' current when the electrode is placed in the external auditory canal or over the ear. At Ca. CI. a sound is heard which gradually diminishes. This sound is variously described as humming, soughing, purring, and sometimes as a distinct ringing. Moderately strong currents (4 to 8 Ma.) are required to produce the effect in most individuals. The An. O. sound is of the same character as the Ca. CI. sound, but not so distinct or long continued. Xo sound is produced on An. CI. or Ca. O.

Testing the galvanic reaction of the auditory nerve is difficult, and attended by many discomforts to the subject of the experiment. Erb uses as the testing electrode a flat electrode, applied over the auricle a little back of the meatus. Brenner used the electrode shown in Fig. 137. The funnel is inserted into the external auditory meatus, and then filled with,, warm water to cause diffusion of the current and

Fig. 137.

prevent injury to the delicate structures in the ear. *Gustatory Nerve.*—A galvanic current in the tongue, or in the vicinity of the gustatory nerve, calls forth a sensation of taste which varies with the pole employed. The cathodic taste is bitterish, while that produced by the anode is of a metallic and somewhat acid character. The sensation sometimes persists for hours after the stimulation. In some persons this " galvanic taste " is developed even though the electrodes are not applied near the mouth or tongue. This sensation is doubtless due to a specific stimulation, direct or reflex, of the gustatory nerve, and not, as some authors have supposed, to electrolysis of the fluids in the mouth. In some persons the cathodic taste cannot be developed, only the anode causing the peculiar sensation. *Olfactory Nerve.* —Weak galvanic currents,.1 to.2 Ma. , produce a peculiar odor when passed through the Schneiderian membrane on Ca. Cl. or An. O.

PHYSIOLOGICAL EFFECTS OF ELECTRIC CURRENTS UPON THE CENTRAL NERVOUS SYSTEM.

Brain.—When a galvanic current is passed transversely through the brain, the electrodes being placed upon the mastoid processes, dizziness is produced, which begins with closure of the circuit, and continues during the passage of the current. The sensation is not merely subjective, but can be demonstrated objectively. The electric vertigo always causes movement of the head toward the side of the anode. On opening the circuit a movement in the opposite direction (toward the cathode) is experienced. Reversal of the current with closed circuit (V. A.) doubles the intensity of the vertigo. The dizziness is produced in the horizontal as well as vertical position. On closing the eyes, or in blind persons, the sensation is experienced as well as with the eyes open, or in those who have good vision. No vertigo is produced when both electrodes are placed on the same side of the head, or when the faradic current is used. This metallic taste, which is very disagreeable to some persons, can be removed by chewing roasted coffee for a few minutes.

Strong galvanic currents sent through the brain also produce co-ordinated ocular movements. The eyeballs move in a jerky manner toward the cathode, and then slowly toward the opposite side, followed by a pendulum-like oscillation from side to side. Stronger currents produce rotatory nystagmus, or fixation of the eyeball toward the side of the cathode.

Confusion of thought, occipital headache, and nausea, or vomiting, sometimes follow the attempts at brain galvanization. Very strong currents have caused fainting and convulsions.

The brain-substance is directly susceptible to galvanic stimulation. Hitzig and Fritsch have demonstrated experimentally that electrical stimulation of certain motor areas in the cerebral cortex causes movements in the appropriate groups of muscles corresponding to the stimulated areas.

Lowenberg states that brain galvanization causes contraction of the vessels in the cathodic area and dilatation in the anodic area. These statements have, however, not been confirmed by any other experimenter.

Spinal Cord.—A galvanic current sent along the spine with the anode at the nape of the neck, and the cathode over the lumbar vertebrae, will sometimes cause contractions in the thighmuscles, as well as sensations (pricking, scalding) in the legs. The benefit derived from galvanism of the spinal cord in certain forms of spinal disease, *e.g.,* tabes dorsalis, chronic myelitis, etc., may be regarded as confirmatory of the experimental results obtained. *Sympathetic Nerve.*—Clinical observation seems to show that electrical stimulation of the superior cervical ganglion of the sympathetic nerve is of benefit in many morbid conditions in which this agent is applied. Careful physiological experiments have failed, however, to give any exact or uniform results from the passage of the current through or in the neighborhood of the ganglion. The method usually adopted to stimulate this ganglion, by the application of one electrode in the auriculomaxillary fossa and the other to the back of the neck, distributes the current over so many important structures that it is impossible to give any definite value to the effect produced upon the ganglion. Most electrotherapeutists, therefore, reject the term "galvanization of the sympathetic," formerly so generally used. The German authors use the expression, "galvanization at the neck," while l)c Watteville proposes the convenient term, "subaural galvanization," which seems to the writer an acceptable phrase, as it simply indicates the point of application of the active electrode. The most usual effects of the galvanic current are a sense of drowsiness and vertigo beginning with the closure, and continuing for some time after the opening, of the circuit; hyperaemia, followed by anaemia of the retina, dilatation of the pupil, diminished blood-pressure and frequency of the pulse, and a general sensation of warmth. None of these effects are constant.

PHYSIOLOGICAL EFFECTS OF ELECTRICAL STIMULATION OF THE THORACIC, ABDOMINAL, AND PELVIC VISCERA.

Heart.—Von Ziemssen has made experiments upon the exposed heart and phrenic nerve in a case where this organ and nerve could be directly reached with the electrodes. The galvanic current increased the force and frequency of the contractions when the electrodes were placed directly upon the heart. The cathode produced more decided effects than the anode. When the current was directed to the ganglionic area, the frequency of the beats was doubled or trebled, but the regularity of pulsation was not interfered with. Strong currents through the chest-walls also increase the frequency of the heart-beats. A current from the spine to the sternum causes cough on closing the circuit.

Direct galvanic stimulation of the phrenic nerve produced in von Ziemssen's experiments the'same series of contractions as are caused in other purely motor nerves. No sensations were produced.

(*Esophagus.*—The muscular coat of this organ contracts promptly upon the application of an electric current through an insulated sound. The faradic current is more prompt in its effects than the galvanic. *Stomach.*—Galvanic stimulation of the stomach produces increased secretion, muscular contraction, and an anaemic condition of the mucous membrane. Faradic currents are often useful in combination with the galvanic. The pyloric extremity of the stomach reacts more promptly to the electrical stimulus than does the cardiac end. When the organ is moderately filled with fluid and gases the contraction is more marked. The stomach can be made to contract either by passing an insulated sound into the organ and stimulating the mucous membrane directly, or through a layer of water with which the organ has been filled; or the electrodes of proper size and shape may be applied to the abdominal walls over the stomach (percutaneous method), or the contractions may be developed by galvanic or faradic stimulation of the vagi. Either of these methods can be adopted for the purpose of physiological experiment, but the percutaneous method is the least troublesome, and apparently effective for therapeutic purposes. *Intestinal Canal.* —Contraction of the lumen of the digestive tube is obtained by limiting the action of the current by means of an insulated intra-intestinal electrode. Percutaneous currents show slight effects, if any, upon the calibre of the tube. Nevertheless, the usefulness of the current in torpor of the intestinal canal cannot be entirely attributed to increased secretion from the mucous layer, but must be clue in a measure to the contractions of the muscles of the intestines, which substitute the ordinary peristaltic movements. *Liver.*—No effects are produced upon this organ by the electric current, so far as our present knowledge extends. *Gallbladder.* — Direct electrization of the gall-bladder will cause contraction of its walls, but no such effect can be demonstrated after the percutaneous application of the current.

Gerhardt, however, advises faradism to the hypochondriac region in cases of catarrhal jaundice, and believes that by the contraction of the muscular coat of the gall-bladder the obstructive plug in the duct can be driven out and the viscus emptied. Von Ziemssen and Bernhardt regard this effect as doubtful, and the latter thinks the favorable result is due to contraction of the abdominal walls, and not to the gall-bladder itself.

Spleen.—The exposed spleen can be made to contract by direct electrization. Contractions can also be produced in this organ by stimulation of the pneumogastric. In certain pathological conditions (malarial enlargement) marked improvement followed percutaneous faradization of the region of the spleen. *Kidneys.*—Experiments upon these organs with the electric current have given negative results. *Urinary Bladder.*—Contractions of this viscus can be produced with both currents. The methods are either percutaneous, or by means of an insulated sound in the bladder and a large abdominal or lumbar electrode. *Urethra.*—The galvanic as well as faradic currents produce contractions of the muscular coat of the urethra. *Uterus.* —The non-pregnant uterus can be stimulated to contraction by direct galvanization and faradization. In the pregnant condition contractions can also be stimulated by application of one electrode to the cervix, and the other to the abdominal wail over the fundus. In post-partum haemorrhage energetic contractions can be produced by intrauterine faradization,—one electrode being applied to the interior of the fundus and the other to the cervix. Menstruation can also be increased by the galvanic current to the uterus. *Ureters.*— The ureters can be made to contract by direct stimulation,—as in physiological experiments,—but in the living subject the electrization of these organs is not practicable.

LOCALIZATION OF THE EFFECTS OF ELECTRIC CURRENTS—MOTOR POINTS OF MUSCLES.

The observations of Duchenne long ago showed that certain points on the surface of the body were apparently "points of election" for the stimulation of certain muscles. R. Remak and von Ziemssen demonstrated that these points correspond to the place of entrance of the motor nerve into the muscle it was intended to stimulate to contraction. They are now called, by all electro-therapeutists, "motor points," after von Ziemssen, who, by his masterly researches, rendered further work on this subject superfluous. In the following account the description of von Ziemssen is closely followed.

Motor Points of the Muscles of the Head, Face, and Neck.— From an examination of Fig. 138, following page, it will be seen that while some of the points where the nerves or muscles can be stimulated are very restricted in size,—are literally "points," —others are lines, in some cases several inches in length. These latter indicate that the respective nerves or muscles can be stimulated to contraction if the exciting electrode is placed at any point along the line. It will be recollected that the galvanic current will give a short, quick contraction or jerk, immediately followed by relaxation unless a very strong current is employed. In order to get a continuous contraction, therefore, the faradic current must be called in requisition. For purposes of diagnosis, indeed, both currents must be used in succession, as will be shown in the next chapter. It will be understood that while in many cases the stimulation of the muscles is spoken of it is usually meant that the stimulation of the nerve causes the muscular contraction. *Facial Nerve.*— The trunk of the facial nerve can be stimulated in the external auditory canal, at the stylo-mastoid foramen, and directly below the external meatus, as exhibited in Effect: To draw the entire half of the face

Figs. 138 and 139.

Rum. comm. pm Mm. triangular «t levator menti

M. levator menti

M. qnadratus menti

M. trbmpnlariii

Rami subcutau. colli N. facial.

Rami cervical, pro Platyamal.

M. steraohyoidcus

M. oinahjroMeiia

M. sternothyroideua.

M. stern ohyoiiIeua aW liadra&c J IX lam rulo *cahn* ,1 *fft S* n,diamj

Fig. 138.—Mgtor Points of The Muscles Of The Head, Face, And Neck. toward the side stimulated. The month and nose are drawn sideways, the eye tightly closed, and the skin thrown into numerous folds. (See Fig. 139.) In some cases of severe facial spasm a similar expression is present.

A

Fig. 139.—Muscles Supplied By The Facial Nerve Stimulated From The Motor Point Below The Meatus.

The post-auricular branch of the facial is reached where it winds around the auricle, as shown in Fig. 138. Effects: To draw the pinna upward and backward, and to depress the scalp posteriorly.

The branches to the stylo-hyoid and digastric muscles can only rarely be stimulated singly. The motor points are situated near to each other, and the muscles usually contract together.

Frg. HI.—Bilateral Contraction Of The Coxeugator Supeecilii Muscles.

The contraction of the attrahens and attollens auriculum is readily stimulated by pressing the electrode on the zygomatic process of the temporal bone, on which the branches of the facial going to those muscles are found. The effect is to draw the auricle upward and forward.

The frontalis muscle is stimulated to contraction through the facial branch which runs superficially from the zygoma over the temporal region. Effect: The skin of the forehead is thrown into numerous transverse folds. (.See Fig. 140.) In old persons the folds are more prominent and numerous. The brows are drawn slightly upward and the folds are curved downward in the centre of the forehead if the contraction is bilateral.

Frg. 142.—Bilateral Contraction-Of The Zyoomaticus Major. The Contraction Of The Orbicularis Palpebrarum Is Also Shown In The Cut.

The expression varies according to the intensity of the contraction from attention to astonishment, surprise, and terror.

The corrugator supercilii is easily isolated at the outer angle of the brow. (See Figs. 138 and 141.) Effects: Flattening and depression of the eyebrows, so that the latter overhang the upper lid. The inner ends of the brows are at the same time drawn upward and inward, throwing the skin into vertical folds over the glabella. The expressions produced are those of reflection, sternness, pain, and anger.

The orbicularis palpebrarum may be stimulated over the malar bone or the parotid gland. (See Fig. 138.) When the nerve is stimulated before its division into its superior and inferior branches the effect is to close the eyelids.

The zygomaticus major can be stimulated to contraction at

Fig. 143.—Contraction or Tfie Zygomaticus Mingr. the posterior inferior border of the malar bone, near the origin of the muscle. Bilateral contraction of this muscle draws the angles of the mouth outward, throws the skin of the cheeks into arc-like folds, and closes the eyes. (See Fig. 142.) The expression caused is that of mirth and laughter, which may be increased to the point of caricature.

The zygomaticus minor can be reached over the junction of the malar bone with the superior maxilla. Its stimulation is always painful on account of the infra-orbital branch of the fifth nerve, which is affected by the current. The effect is to raise the upper lip and draw it outward, causing an expression of dissatisfaction or pain. (See Fig. 143.)

The levator labii superioris is difficult to isolate, but can sometimes be picked out on the side of the nose near the motor point for the zygomaticus minor. Its contraction raises the upper lip on the stimulated side perpendicularly, and sometimes exposes the teeth. (See Fig. 144.)

Stimulation of the levator labii superioris alaeque nasi, on

Fig. 144—Contraction Of The Levator Labii Superioris Proprius. the side of the bridge of the nose, produces, like the preceding, a weeping or whining expression. (See Fig. 145.)

In order to produce complete contraction of the orbicularis oris four electrodes are necessary, one applied to each of the motor points, shown in Fig. 138, where the branches of the nerve enter the muscle. It is, perhaps, better on the whole to stimulate the muscle directly. Effects: Its complete contraction produces projection of the lips (pouting), and throws the skin and mucous membrane into fine folds.

The buccinator may be stimulated at the inner border of

Fig. 145.—Contraction Of The Levator Labii Superioris Al2eo.ue Nasi. the massetcr. Effects: The mouth is drawn to one side mid the cheek is pressed against the gums and teeth. (See Fig. 146.)

The triangularis menti may he isolated near the angle of the jaw, or may be caused to contract jointly with the levator menti by stimulating the common branch of the facial running to these muscles before its division. Effects: It draws the anijle of the mouth and the outer half of the, lower lip downward and outward, widening but not opening the mouth.

The quadratus menti is best stimulated directly, as it is difficult to isolate the nerve going to it. Effect: To draw the respective sides of the lower lip downward and outward, pressing it against the teeth. (See Fig. 147.)

The levator menti may sometimes be stimulated by application of the electrode over the nerve after it branches off from the nerve supplying this muscle and the triangularis, but it is usually better to apply the electrode upon the muscle itself just at the inner edge of the quadratus. Bilateral contraction of the levator menti causes flattening of the chin, and partial ectropium of the lower lip. The expression produced is that of contemptuous haughtiness. (See Figs. 148 and 149.) Von Ziemssen says, with ill-concealed sarcasm, that this muscle may be considered the interpreter of exalted self-consciousness in scientists, officials, and aristocrats. He calls it the "Geheimraths-muskel," — privy-councillor's muscle.

The masseter and temporal muscles can be made to con

Fig. 148.—Contraction of The Levator Menti (profile View). tract only by direct muscular stimulation, as the nervous supply is too deeply situated to be reached from the surface. The masseter can be stimulated in the sigmoid notch of the lower jaw; the temporal by one electrode on the anterior and the other on the posterior division of the muscle. Effect: Strong closure of the mouth and chattering of the teeth.

Contraction of the lingual muscles can be produced by unilateral application of an electrode, on either side, above, or below.

The velum of the palate can be drawn upward so as to close the posterior nares, by using two electrodes.

The uvula can be made to disappear almost entirely by pressing a fine electrode lightly against its base. The azygos muscle contracts and the entire uvula seems to shrink up, leaving only a small knob-like projection.

By pressing an electrode against the internal wall of the pharynx the constrictors can be readily brought into play.

Fig. 149.—Bilateral Contraction Of The Levator Menti (front View).

The platysma myoides receives its nerve-supply from the descending facial and the cervical plexus. In order to produce complete contraction both electrodes must be used, one being placed over the cervical branch at the middle of the sternocleido-mastoid and the other over the branches of the facial nerve. In Fig. 138 these points are indicated as "rami cervical, pro platysmat.," and "rami subcutan. colli n. facial." Effect: the depression between the lower jaw and the clavicle is flattened, and the skin thrown into vertical folds. The lower lip is drawn downward, and if the current is strong the teeth are exposed. The expression produced is that of wrath, fear, and horror, especially if the frontalis and corrugatores supercilii are caused to contract at the same time.

The sterno-cleido-mastoid can be stimulated to contraction at the middle of the upper half of the muscle. One-sided contraction of this muscle causes twisting of the head toward the opposite side of the body and the head is bent downward sideways, as is well shown in Fig. 150.

Fig. 150.—One-sided Contraction Of The Sterno-cleido-mastoid.

Bilateral contraction causes projection of the face, with elevation of the chin and bending of the cervical spine.

The trapezius muscle is easily stimulated to contraction by placing the electrode over the external branch of the spinal accessory nerve, which can be readily reached from a point near the insertion of the sterno-cleido-mastoid, running over the upper portion of this muscle, and outward toward the shoulder, as shown in Fig. 138.

The effect of bilateral stimulation is shown in Fig. 151. The shoulders are raised and the scapulae drawn toward the spine. The skin of the neck is thrown into large folds.

The levator anguli scapulae is supplied by a branch from the fourth cervical nerve, which can be isolated with a fine electrode a little below the motor point for the trapezius. Effect: To raise the inner angle of the scapula, and draw it inward and forward. The superior and inferior clavicular spaces are converted into deep sulci and the clavicle rendered extremely prominent.

The sterno-thyroid, omo-hyoid, and sterno-hyoid may be reached at the anterior border of the sterno-cleido-mastoid near its middle. The two latter can also be stimulated between the two points of origin of the sterno-cleido-mastoid muscle.

The phrenic nerve is found at the outer border of the sternocleido-mastoid, in front of the scalenus anticus and above the omo-hyoid. Effect: Rapid contraction of the diaphragm, projection of the belly, and forcible inspiration. As faradization of the phrenic nerve is a recognized procedure in suspended respiration, it is important that it should be frequently practiced in order that the method may be familiar should the physician be suddenly required to employ it. The electrodes (bilaterally) should be pressed inward firmly behind the clavicular portion of the sterno-cleido-mastoid.

The isolated electrical stimulation of the laryngeal muscles is extremely difficult even to the expert laryngoscopist. Percutaneously, the crico-thyroids can be thrown into strong contraction by applying the electrodes on either side of the cricothyroid ligament.

Stimulation of the pneumogastric nerve is uncertain, although a number of authors assert its practicability. Duchenne used an oesophageal electrode, while others apply the electrode at the inner border of the sterno-cleido-niastoid muscle, immediately below the omo-hyoid muscle.

The brachial plexus is easily stimulated as a whole, but the isolated stimulation of single nerves is often difficult. The three heavy bars on the side of the neck show the area for stimulating the plexus. (See Fig. 138.)

The posterior thoracic nerve is reached near the spinal accessory at the border of the trapezius. Its stimulation causes contraction of the rhomboid and serratus posticus superior, drawing the scapula toward the spine and upward, and slightly raising the upper ribs.

The lateral thoracic nerve is stimulated above the clavicle near the border of the trapezius. Effect: contraction of the serratus magnus, drawing the scapula forward.

The anterior thoracic is best reached below the clavicle and at the upper border of the pectoralis major muscle. Its stimulation causes the upper arm to be drawn forcibly against the chest.

At the upper end of the middle bar (Fig. 138), showing the surface for stimulating the brachial plexus, is a point whence a group of muscles consisting of the deltoid, biceps, brachialis anticus, and supinator longus can be stimulated to contraction.

This was first indicated by Erb and called by him the supraclavicular point. It is now generally known as "Erb's point." *Motor Points of the Upper Extremity.*—In many persons the axillary nerve can be reached at a point just above the clavicle, and a little external to the surface for the brachial plexus. Stimulation of this nerve produces strong contraction of the deltoid muscle.

The musculo-cutaneous nerve is found in the depression between the coraco-brachialis and the biceps, or between the two heads of the latter. (See Fig. 152.) Stimulation of this

N. muiculo-cutan. M. bicepa.

nerve causes contraction of the biceps and brachialis anticus muscles, flexing the forearm.

The biceps alone is stimulated a little below the point above mentioned, and the brachialis anticus about the middle of the arm.

The median nerve is found along the entire length of the bicipital groove, but can be best stimulated at the lower third of the humerus, where it may be pressed against the bone. Its stimulation causes contraction in the pronator quadratus and teres, flexor carpi radialis, palmaris longus, flexor sublimis and profundus, the muscles of the ball of the thumb, and the three first lumbricalcs. Effects: Strong pronation of the forearm, flexing the hand toward the radial side, flexing the fingers, and opposition of the thumb.

In the forearm the median is found superficially one inch above the wrist-joint between the tendons of the flexor radialis and the palmaris longus. Effects: Abduction of the thumb with strong spasm and slight flexion of the first phalanges of the index and middle fingers, and generally of the ring-finger (Fig. 153).

The flexor sublimis and profundus digitorum cannot be stimulated alone through their nerves, but can be directly caused to contract at the points marked in Fig. 154. The flexor carpi

Fig. 153.—Effect Of Stimulation Of Median Nerve In The Forearm. radialis and palmaris longus can be stimulated at points indicated. The flexor radialis and palmaris longus can best be stimulated through the nerves at the points shown in the figure (154). The branches to the pronator quadratus and the flexor pollicis longus cannot be stimulated owing to their deep location. The ulnar nerve can be stimulated throughout its course from the axilla to the elbow, but the best point at which to apply the electrode is the groove between the olecranon and the internal condyle of the humerus. Faradic stimulation of the nerve at this point produces pain in the area of distribution of the branch to the palmaris longus and the branches to the dorsal and volar surfaces of the hands, as well as contractions of the flexor carpi ulnaris, flexor profundus, palmaris brevis, the interossei, lumbricalcs, adductor pollicis, and the little-finger muscles.

The motor root for the flexor ulnaris can sometimes be isolated at its entrance into the muscle one inch below the internal condyle. The muscle can be directly stimulated by applying the electrodes immediately upon it. It draws the hand toward the ulnar side.

Fig. 154.—Motor Points Op Forearm.

In the lower part of its course the ulnar nerve is easily found on the radial side of the tendon of the flexor carpi ulnaris (Fig. 154). Its stimulation produces contraction of the muscles of the hand above mentioned, and causes the hollowing of the hand, adduction of the thumb, flexion and opposition of the little finger, and moderate flexion of the remaining fingers at the metacarpo-phalangeal joints.

Fig. 155.—Contraction Of The Opponent Pollicis.

The abductor, flexor, and opponens minimi digiti are all three found in close proximity near the ulnar border of the palm, the latter being farthest inward and forward. (See Fig. 154.)

Fig. 156—Motor Points Of The Arm. (extensor Surface.)

The motor point for the palmaris brevis is found a little farther back and inward.

The muscles of the ball of the thumb—abductor pollicis brevis, opponens pollicis, and flexor pollicis brevis—are easily stimulated through the nerves. Fig. 154 shows the motor points. The effect of contraction of the opponens pol?licis is shown in Fig. 155.

Pig. 157.—Motor Points Of The Extensor Surface Of Forearm And Hand.

The lumbricales are reached at the points indicated in Fig. 154. Their stimulation produces slight flexion of the first phalanges and twisting of the fingers toward the ulnar side of the hand. The fourth and fifth lumbricales of violin-players give a specially good reaction on account of the development of these muscles in such persons.

The other palmar muscles are difficult to isolate and stimulate singly to contraction.

The radial nerve can be stimulated at a point midway between the insertion of the deltoid and the external condyles of the humerus (Fig. 156). Its stimulation causes pain in the area of distribution of the superficial radial to the dorsal surfaces of the fingers, and contraction of the supinator brevis, extensor carpi radialis longus and brevis, extensor carpi ulnaris, extensores communis, indicis, minimi digiti, pollicis longus and brevis, and adductor pollicis. The effect is supination of the forearm, with extension of the hand and thumb and extension of the first phalanges of the fingers, the remaining phalanges being partly flexed.

Fig. 158.—Stimulation Of The Abductor Pollicis Longus.

The extensor carpi radialis longior can only be stimulated by direct electrization, as the nerve is too deeply situated to respond to the current.

The supinator brevis, extensor carpi radialis brevis, extensor carpi ulnaris, anconeus, and extensor communis are likewise only accessible to direct electrical stimulation. (See Figs. 156, 157.)

The abductor pollicis longus is stimulated about midway between the elbow and wrist near the radial border of the forearm (Fig. 157). Its action is to abduct the thumb, leaving the last phalanx partly flexed (Fig. 158).

The extensor indicis is reached a little above the point for the abductor pollicis, and between these two is a common motor point for both muscles.

The extensor minimi digiti can rarely be stimulated alone through the nerve, but contraction can be produced by sending the current directly through the muscle. The point is a little above the middle of the forearm near the ulnar border.

Motor Points of the Trunkal Muscles.—The action of the intercostal muscles is to raise the ribs during inspiration. However, owing. to the superposition of other muscles, the former cannot be isolated and their actions separately studied in the normal condition. By pressing the electrode firmly against the lower border of the ribs the muscles for that interspace will be thrown into contraction.

The motor points for the recti muscles of the abdomen are four or five in number. Simultaneous stimulation of all these points causes flattening of the abdomen. When those above the umbilicus are alone stimulated the abdominal wall is drawn upward; when those below are stimulated the wall is drawn downward.

The external oblique muscle has four or five points laterally above the umbilicus. (See Fig. 159). The action is to flatten the lateral abdominal walls.

The transversalis muscle of the. abdomen can be stimulated at the anterior border of the quadratus lumborum just above the crest of the ilium.

The internal oblique is reached above the anterior superior iliac spine and just in front of the point for the transversalis.

The latissimus dorsi can easily be stimulated directly, but the points of nerve-supply are extremely difficult to find.

Motor Points of the Lower Extremity.— The motor points of the lower extremity are usually found over the muscles themselves, and contraction of the latter can be most easily produced by direct stimulation. The principal branch of the crural nerve which supplies the extensor muscles of the thigh can be isolated at the inner border of the rectus femoris about the middle of the thigh. Its stimulation causes contraction of all the extensors of the thigh (quadriceps femoris).

The rectus can be stimulated at a point a little external to the last. The electrode is pushed under the inner border of the muscle. The vastus externus may be stimulated through two points on the outer border of the thigh a few inches above the knee.

The cruraeus is found at the inner border of the sartorius at the junction of the middle and lower thirds of the thigh, and the vastus internus along the inner border of the sartorius in the lower third. The sartorius is stimulated at the apex of Scarpa's triangle. Two electrodes should be used, one at the point mentioned and the other on the lower half of the muscle.

The tensor vaginae femoris (tensor fasciae latae) derives its nerve-supply from two sources, the superior gluteal and the crural nerves. The muscle presents two motor points, one near the outer border of the thigh directly outward from the exit of the crural nerve, and the other somewhat lower and farther inward. (See Fig. 160.)

The obturator nerve can be found over the obturator foramen. Its stimulation produces adduction of the thigh. Of the branches of the obturator nerve, those going to the adductores brevis, longus, and magnus, and to the gracilis, may sometimes be singly stimulated to contraction.

The sciatic nerve (Fig. 161) is reached with a strong cur rent and large electrode applied between the trochanter major and the tuber ischii. Its stimulation produces contraction in the flexor muscles of the leg and foot, and pain in the area of distribution of the sensitive fibres.

The heads of the biceps are each supplied with a branch of the sciatic nerve. That going to the long head is reached in the middle of the thigh, just under the fleshy part of the buttock. The short head is reached lower down and nearer the outer border of the thigh.

The semi-tendinosus and semi-membranosus muscles may be stimulated at the same height as the long head of the biceps, but nearer the inner border of the thigh.

Fig. 163.—Motor Points Of Back Of Leo And Inner Border Of The Foot.

The peronei, tibialis anticus, extensor communis longior et brevior and extensor hallucis longus are stimulated to contraction through the peroneal nerve, which is reached where it crosses the posterior aspect of the head of the fibula.

The tibialis anticus can also be isolated through a motor point about three and a half inches below the head of the fibula. (See Fig. 162.) Its stimulation produces strong dorsal flexion of the foot, with a slight outward turn.

The extensor communis longus is found parallel to the tibialis anticus, but a little farther outward.

The posterior leg-muscles can be stimulated to contraction by placing the electrode over the posterior tibial nerve in the popliteal space. The nervous branches to the individual muscles are difficult to isolate, but the motor points for intramuscular stimulation are indicated in Figs. 162 and 163.

CHAPTER II.

Electro-diagnosis.

Both the faradic and galvanic currents are used for diagnostic purposes in pathological conditions of nerves and muscles.

When the faradic current is employed it is of little consequence which pole is used, as the reaction of the nerve and muscle is the same in quality for both poles. The secondary spiral acts, however, with greater intensity, and is for this reason usually employed.

On the other hand, when the galvanic or constant current is used, the selection of the pole to which the testing electrode is attached is of the greatest importance. This will be readily appreciated when it is borne in mind how differently the two poles act upon nerve and muscle, or upon the organs of special sense, in their normal condition.

The diagnosis of morbid conditions of nerves and muscles by means of the electric current demands certain special qualities in the physician that will have been appreciated perhaps by those who have read the preceding sections of this work. The electro-diagnostician must have a good practical knowledge of the apparatus employed, and he must be familiar with the location of the various motor points of muscles, and of the effects produced when these are stimulated in their normal condition.

The pathological conditions which modify the normal reactions and the nature of these modifications will be described in this chapter.

In order to permit the comparison of different observations the same apparatus—batteries, electrodes, galvanometers, rheostats, etc.—should always be used. Care must be taken that the connections in the circuit are tight and without insulation, and, unless previously determined, the anode and cathode should be found by experiment and appropriately marked.

The electrodes most suitable for testing are the so-called "normal" electrode of Erb and the "unit" electrode of Stintzing. The former has an area of ten square centimetres and the latter three square centimetres. With the latter finer work in isolating nerves lying close together can be done, but its use requires an exactness of anatomical knowledge which is not very common. Hence, for practical purposes the normal electrode of Erb will give greater satisfaction.

The testing electrode should have a key for closing and opening the circuit conveniently in the handle. More complicated electrodes, such as contain commutator and rheostat in the handle, are not desirable, since they are liable to get out of order, and are either cumbersome or untrustworthy.

As the indifferent electrode, the large, "indifferent" electrode of Erb may be used. The size of this is not very important, but it should be sufficiently large to diffuse the current so as to cause no reaction at the point where it is applied. The point of application should always be the same, the sternum being generally selected by electro-therapeutists on account of convenience, absence of points of irritation, and equability of surface.

In testing the irritability of nerves and muscles for diagnostic purposes, a regular programme should be adopted and always followed. This soon becomes habitual, and errors and omissions more rarely occur than when an irregular course is followed.

Supposing the case presented for diagnosis were a one-sided lesion of the facial nerve, the electrical reactions of the nerve and muscles of the *sound* side should first be tested, beginning with the faradic current and then testing with the galvanic current. After determining *seriatim* the electrical reactions, both faradic and galvanic, on the sound side, and entering them upon an appropriate record-blank, the same course should be gone through with on the diseased or injured side, following the same order of proceeding.

The reason for using the faradic current first is this: The passage of the induced current has little, if any, influence upon resistance (or conductivity) of the epidermis, while the galvanic current invariably reduces this resistance after passing a short time. It is evident that when the resistance is diminished a weaker current would produce the reaction tested for in the nerves and muscles. This would cause confusion in the records, and the practitioner would not be able to compare the reactions given from day to day, or week to week. Hence, the importance of having a regular scheme or programme for electro-diagnostic examinations which should be adhered to in daily practice.

In testing with the faradic current the secondary coil should be used. The strength of current is noted upon the scale affixed to the sledge induction apparatus. This scale is usually divided into millimetres, and indicates the distance to which the outer coil is made to slide over the inner. The German authors call this distance "Rollenabstand," and indicate it by the symbol Ra. We may call it "coil distance," and use C. D. as a symbol. Thus, in the apparatus used by the writer the total coil distance possible is 150 mm. In other words, when the outer or secondary coil is drawn completely out so as to uncover the primary coil throughout its whole extent the distance between the beginning of the primary and of the secondary coils is 150 mm. This point of total separation is the zero point of the secondary current. In order to strengthen the secondary current the outer spiral is shoved over the inner coil, and as the distance is diminished the strength of current is increased. When the primary current of the induction coil is employed the weakest current is obtained with the C. D. at zero; in other words, when the outer coil completely covers the inner one. When the secondary current is employed this condition of things is reversed, and when the coils completely cover each other, when the C. D. is 0, the current is at its greatest strength.

The following tabular presentation will perhaps make this a little clearer:—
PRIMARY CURRENT. SECONDARY CURRENT.
C. D. 0 mm. = weakest current.
C. D. 150 mm. = strongest current.
C. P. 0 mm. = strongest current.
C. D. 150 mm. = weakest current.

On the instrument used by the writer there is a double scale, which is read so as to indicate the weakest current by 0 mm. and the strongest 150 mm. for each current. This simplifies the recording of results, but to make the record absolutely exact the number of millimetres coil distance should have a letter or symbol appended indicating whether the current is primary or secondary. Thus, if contraction were produced by a current of 25 mm. coil distance of the secondary current it might be written 25 mm. C. D. s. If, on the other hand, the current was the primary one and the coil distance 30 mm., we should write 30 mm. C. D. p.

The practical difference in the effects of the induction machine deserves the most careful attention of the physician who busies himself at all with electricity. Careless handling of the electrodes when the C. D. indicates the maximum strength of current may give a shock that is not only painful but under some conditions dangerous.

The strength of the induced current depends upon the battery, the number and size of the spirals in the coil, the size and resistance of the wire, the insulation, the length and thickness of the coil, and certain other conditions more fully pointed out in the first part of this work. (See page 87.)

It will be evident, on careful consideration of the conditions governing the construction and operating of the induction coil, that it is extremely difficult to construct two instruments of identical qualities as regards strength of current, etc. Hence differences, slight or great, are always to be assumed between any two induction apparatuses. For this reason the results obtained from one instrument are not exactly comparable with another. The record of the C. D. in testing the reaction in any case is simply for the purpose of comparing the results obtained with subsequent tests in the same case and on the same nerve or muscle.

Even if the instruments were standardized so as to admit of comparison of observations, the varying resistance of the skin and other tissues of different individuals, and of the same individual at different times, would be an effective bar to the exact comparison of results unless the resistance of the skin in each case were likewise determined and noted, with the size, position, and degree of moisture of the electrodes used.

The desirability, however, of having some sort of standard induction apparatus with which others could be compared has led the Electrical Congress of Paris, of 1881, to suggest a normal or standard apparatus of the following dimensions. The galvanic generator is a single Daniell's cell. The various parts of the apparatus are as follows:—

Primary Coil. Secondary Coil.
Length of spool (excluding wooden frame), 88 mm. 65 mm.
Diameter of spool,.... 36" 68"
Diameter of wire,.... 1" 0.25"
Number of turns of wire,...300 5000
Layers of wire, 4 28'

Resistance, primary coil, about 1.5 Siemens' units; secondary coil, about 300 Siemens' units.

When this standard machine is used the same C. D. should give approximately the same results, other conditions being equal.

Stintzing has endeavored to determine the average faradic irritability for different nerves, in order to furnish a standard of what may be called a "normal reaction" for comparison. By using the same coil and battery and his "unit electrode" of three square centimetres contact surface he constructed the following table of average values in coil distance:—

Mathematically expressed, he finds the density of current (D) equal to the coil distance in millimetres divided by the electrode of three square centimetres contact surface, or, according to the equation, x mm. C. D. 52 cm.

The following table of the average faradic irritability is from Stintzing. The notation is on the German scale, using the secondary current. The second column of figures gives the values translated into readings on the double scale, as found on some American-made coils (0 mm. C. D. = 0 current), the maximum length of the scale being 150 mm.

It must be remembered that the results obtained from two different instruments cannot be compared with each other, but every one can determine on one or more cases the divergence of bis own instrument from the above table of normal averages, and use the same as a factor for correcting his observations.

In like manner to the above, Stintzing has determined the galvanic irritability of certain nerves to be used as standards for comparison. The current strength is indicated in milliamperes.
0 mm. C. D. = maximum current. 150 mm. C. D. = 0 current, f o mm. C. D. = 0 current. 150 mm. C. D. = maximum current.

The formula for computing these results is similar to the one employed in determining the faradic irritability, using the number of milliamperes as a numerator in the equation:—

It will be noticed that the different nerves react differently to the galvanic and faradic currents.

Lewandowski also gives a brief table, showing the current required for producing all the phenomena of the complete law of contraction, noting the current in milliamperes. The testing electrode was the "normal electrode" of Erb (102 cm.):—

The density of the current is proportional to its strength and inversely proportional to the area of the electrode at the point of application to the surface of the body. It must not be forgotten, however, that we cannot by any means at present at our command determine the density of the current at its point of entry into the nerve; hence, while measurements of current strength, as in the preceding tables, are of a certain value as guides in practice, they teach us nothing of the current density required to stimulate the nerve itself to contraction.

The beginner in electro-diagnosis should not operate too long on the same nerve at a sitting, because the reduction of resistance resulting from prolonged passage of the galvanic current apparently increases the irritability of the nerves, and is hence liable to lead to incorrect conclusions. The motor points should first be found and determined

with the faradic current and marked on the skin with an indelible pencil, in order to render renewed search for them unnecessary. The patient should always be examined in the same position, which should be the horizontal in most cases.

In addition to the clinical history of the case, the electrical irritability in cases where this is determined should be entered in a special record. The form devised by von Ziemssen, and in use in the hospital in Munich, seems to be practically arranged. Each page of the record is divided into six spaces, each of which can be appropriated for a nerve or muscle tested. At the right hand at the top of the sheet is a space for the name, and at the left a space for the diagnosis. Above the upper line the form is divided into three divisions, the centre one being for the name of the nerve or muscle and the size of the testing electrode, while the side divisions are marked "right" and "left" respectively. The body of the form is divided into six columns, the first being for the date, the second and sixth being for remarks descriptive of the nature of the contraction produced by the galvanic current, sensibility, mechanical irritability, etc. The upper division of the third and fifth columns gives the coil distance at which faradic irritability is manifested, while the lower division of the same columns shows the number of milliamperes of current required to produce the galvanic contraction formula.

Various forms of charts are also used by electro-therapeutists to record graphically the reactions of nerves and muscles. The following are from Erb's classical work on "ElectroTherapeutics." The references at the side of the chart show with sufficient definiteness the meaning of the different curves.

Fig. l&i.—Cases Of Paralysis,-with Early Return of Voluntary Motion. 10 11 21
Motility.
Galv. muscular reaction,
Faradic muscular reaction.
Galv. and farad, reaction of nerve.
Motility
Galv. muscular reaction

Fari.li.. muscular reaction
Galr. and farad7 reaction of nerve.
Th asterisk shows the date of reappearance of the power of voluntary motion. The figures at the top of the chart indicate the number of week the case is under observation.

The qualitative differences of galvanic reaction (It. 1).) can also be shown by means of charts, several of which are shown in Fig. 165. The first tracing shows the relations between the C'a. CI. C. (A'O and the An. CI. C. *(An)* in the healthy nerve; the second shows the degeneration of the nerve and reversal of the law of contraction, An. CI. C. *(An)* being much stronger than Ca. CI. C. *(Kn)*, which is almost inappreciable. The third tracing shows the effect of a stronger current in the same case.

The alterations of electrical irritability of nerve and muscle produced by disease may be classed under three heads, viz:— 1. *Quantitative,* or an increase, diminution, or total disappearance of electrical irritability to one or both currents.

2. *Qualitative,* consisting in a modification in kind of the normal reactions of nerve and muscle to electric currents. This is the so-called "reaction of degeneration." 3. *Mixed,* or combinations of quantitative and qualitative variations of irritability. This class may also be included under the consideration of reaction of degeneration.

These three classes of modified electrical irritability will now be discussed more in detail.

I. QUANTITATIVE CHANGES IN ELECTRICAL IRRITABILITY.
Increased Electrical Irritability.—Increase of faradic irritability is present in tabes dorsalis and tetany. The contraction follows the passage of a much weaker current than is required to produce contraction normally. Stintzing's standards of faradic irritability may be used for comparison.

Galvanic irritability is increased in the following diseases: Fresh hemiplegias with phenomena of motor irritation, spasms, contractures, beginning acute and subacute myelitis, hemichorea, tetany, various stages of tabes dorsalis, progressive muscular atrophy (considerable increase in non-atrophic and perfectlyfunctioning motor areas), peripheral paralysis, early stage of rheumatic and facial paralysis, and beginning neuritis.

Diminished Electrical Irritability.—This is very frequently present in the most varied affections of the motor apparatus. The faradic irritability may vary greatly at different portions of the same nerve. No satisfactory explanation can yet be given of this phenomenon. Thus, Erb found in one case the difference of C. D. to rise from the normal difference of 10 to 20 mm. to 42 to oo mm. In another case the difference was even greater.

Faradic and galvanic irritability are usually diminished in the same proportion, although in some cases the faradic increase is combined with galvanic decrease, and *vice verm.* Diseases in which the electrical irritability is diminished arc: progressive myelitis, advanced tabes dorsalis, spastic spinal paralysis, multiple sclerosis, brain tumors, advanced cerebral hemiplegia (on the paralyzed side), progressive bulbar paralysis, in melancholia and paralytic dementia, progressive muscular atrophy, true and pseudo-hypertrophy of muscles, acute and chronic poliomyelitis, multiple neuritis, amyotrophic lateral sclerosis, writers' cramp, muscular atrophies from inaction of muscles, toxic paralyses (arsenical, alcoholic, carbonic oxide, chloroform poisoning, etc.), and in the paralyses following infectious diseases.

Some authors describe a form of decreased electrical irritability which has been appropriately named, "reaction of exhaustion." When present it is found that a reaction, produced by a certain strength of current, cannot be reproduced without increasing the current. The discharge of nerve-force responding to a certain definite irritation fails on repetition of the irritation of the same intensity. The nerve or muscle seems to have been. exhausted by the first contraction, and only by increasing the strength of the current can a second contraction be produced. This phenomenon has been observed in cerebral paralysis, progressive muscular atrophy, paralysis agitans, anterior poliomyelitis, brain tumors, etc.

II. QUALITATIVE CHANGES IN ELECTRICAL IRRITABILITY.
Reaction of Degeneration (R. D.J.—Under this designation, first introduced by Erb, is understood a modification of electrical irritability which is characteristic of certain morbid conditions of nerve and muscle, and which, when present, is pathognomonic of certain diseases, and hence becomes an important diagnostic sign.

The phenomena of the reaction of degeneration are comprised in the following modifications of irritability:— *a.* Disappearance or diminution of the nervous irritability to both galvanic and faradic currents.

b. Disappearance of faradic and increase of galvanic irritability of the muscle, generally associated with increased mechanical irritability. *c.* Tardy, delayed contraction of the stimulated muscle, instead of the quick, lightning-like contraction of the normal muscle. *d.* Appearance of certain decided modifications of the normal formula of contraction.

The essential feature of the reaction of degeneration seems to be the tardy contraction of the muscle in place of the quick, lightning-like contraction (or jerk") of the normal muscle. This is due to the fact, as pointed out by von Ziemssen, that in the degenerative changes in nerve and muscle following peripheral paralysis no reaction occurs to momentary stimuli, but when the stimulation is prolonged contraction slowly follows.

The individual phenomena making up the reaction of degeneration are best studied in severe traumatic or rheumatic paralyses. Supposing the case to be one of ordinary facial paralysis,—neuritic, rheumatic, or Bell's paralysis (Fig. 166),— the electrical reactions would be somewhat as follows:— 1. In the beginning of the paralysis there is sometimes a slight increase of the *nervous* irritability, the response to both currents being more prompt on the paralyzed than on the healthy side, but alter the second or third day both the faradic and galvanic irritability of the affected *nerve* and its branches decrease, so that on each succeeding day stronger currents are required to produce contractions. Between the eighth and twelfth days the electrical irritability of the *nerve* to both currents disappears entirely.

2. About the same time the paralyzed *muscles* gradually lose their *faradic* irritability, but the *galvanic* irritability rapidly increases, so that very slight currents are required to produce contractions. For example, if the muscles in the area of distribution of the facial nerve on the unaffected side require a current of 4 milliamperes to produce the minimum contraction, a current of only 0.4 milliamperes is necessary to produce contraction on the paralyzed side. Cases even occur where contractioiis can be produced in the paralyzed muscles while testing the muscles on the healthy side.

This condition of hyper-irritability of the muscle to the galvanic current usually lasts several weeks and then gradually subsides, until, finally, the muscle also fails to react to the stimulation of either current.

3. Coincidently with the increase of galvanic irritability there appears a change in the mode of contraction which is extremely characteristic. The normal reaction to the current is, as is well known, a sharp, flash-like jerk, the muscle immediately becoming relaxed until the current is broken, when an equally sharp "opening contraction" occurs. In the reaction of degeneration, this quick, jerky contraction is changed into a sluggish, tardy, drawing-up of the muscle-substance. This is the essential and jwthognomonic feature of the reaction of degeneration. When absent, there is no reaction of degeneration, no matter what other modification of the normal law of contraction may be present.

During the stage of galvanic hyper-irritability there is also an increase of the mechanical irritability of the muscle.

4. The change in the normal formula of contraction, which usually, though not always, appears in conjunction with the stage of hyper-irritability, is very remarkable. The anodal closing contraction, which is only produced in the normal condition by a current considerably stronger than that to which the muscle responds when the cathode is used, responds gradually to a weaker and weaker current, until, finally, it is excited by a current little if any stronger, or sometimes even weaker, than that producing the cathodal closing contraction. The anodal opening contraction and cathodal opening contraction also approach nearer to the cathodal closing contraction than in the normal condition.

In the typical form of R. T)., therefore, the normal formula of contraction (seep. 149), viz., Ca. Cl. C; An. O.C. ; An. Cl. C.; Ca. Te.; Ca. O. C, is changed as follows: An. Cl. C.; Ca. Cl. C.; An. O. C.; Ca. O. C, or some modification of this formula. (See Fig. 165.)

Alter four to six weeks the galvanic hyper-irritability gradually diminishes until eventually the reaction to the strongest current is almost or quite lost. The An. Cl. C. is the last to disappear. If the injured or diseased nerve is regenerated, voluntary power, the normal formula of contraction as well as the flash-like character of the contraction are gradually reestablished. On the other hand, when the degeneration of the nerve is complete, the contractility of the muscles is never

Fig. lfiT.—Oi.d Facial Paralysis, Showing Complete Loss Of Mcscn.ar Contractility On The Paralyzed Side. (After Oowers.)

restored, and years after electrical stimulation is limited in its effects to one side, as shown in Fig. 167.

When regeneration of the nerve occurs the trophic activity is first manifested in the improved nutrition of the muscles; then follows a return of voluntary power, and finally restoration of the electrical irritability.

The muscular irritability to both currents returns gradually, the slow, tardy contractions giving place to the fulgurant ones and the normal formula of contraction being re-established.

The above-described modifications of the normal electrical irritability of the paralyzed nerve and muscle are due to certain changes in these structures, which have been experimentally studied by Erb, Neumann, Leegaard, Sigmund Mayer, and Gessler. The histological changes found in the nerves consist of a granular, lumpy degeneration of the medullary sheath beginning within a few days of the lesion to the nerve. This is followed by softening of the axis cylinder, which is substituted by protoplasmic masses. This is accompanied by nuclear proliferation of the sheath of Schwann and cellular accumulation in the neurilemma, from which young connective tissue is developed. The entire nerve is permeated with this newly-formed connective tissue. After a time, in case regeneration is possible, the normal condition of the nerve is gradually restored, the regeneration beginning at the periphery and not at the central point of the lesion. The newly-formed connective tissue is, however, not entirely absorbed, but remains to a greater or less degree as an evidence of the nutritive disturbance which has taken place in the nerve.

The changes in the muscle consist of simple atrophy of the primitive fasciculi of the muscular fibres, with occasional areas of fatty degeneration, excessive nuclear proliferation, cell accumulation in the interstitial connective tissue, and hyperplasia of the latter. This condition may become permanent, and the muscle then appears as a thin band of connective tissue with muscular fibres disseminated through its substance.

When restoration of function occurs the new-formed connective tissue is reabsorbed, but the normal state of the muscle is never entirely restored.

The motor end-plates in the muscle are the last structures to yield to the degenerative processes and the first to be restored in structure and function.

The histological changes in the paralyzed nerve and muscle explain the phenomena of the reaction of degeneration. The solution of continuity at the point where the lesion of the nerve is situated abolishes the power of transmission of voluntary impulses, as well as of proximal electrical stimulation of the nerve.

The diminution of electrical irritability beyond the lesion in the nerve is due to the progressive degeneration of the nervestructure. The disappearance of the faradic irritability in the muscle, as well as the sluggish contraction of the latter under the galvanic current, is due to degeneration of the muscle-substance itself, for the phenomena of the It. D. are present in the muscle at a time when the nerve-terminations have not yet undergone degeneration.

The researches of Gessler upon nerve degeneration in coldblooded animals appear to show that the true R. D., viz. , tardy contractions upon galvanic stimulation with no response upon faradic stimulation, is entirely due to muscular degeneration. While in these animals complete nerve degeneration occurred, muscular degeneration as well as the phenomenon of reaction of degeneration remained absent.

The final disappearance of galvano-muscular irritability is an evidence of the increased atrophy of the muscular fibre and the excessive interstitial connective-tissue hyperplasia.

The electrical irritability of the nerve and muscle does not return coincidently with the power of conveying motor impulses. The former function requires a more advanced stage of nerve regeneration than the latter. This discrepancy between the duration of voluntary and electrical suspension of irritability of nerve and muscle is explained by the assumption that the *transmission* of an impression from the nerve-centre—in other words, the *conductivity* of the nerve—requires a less perfect organ than the origination of an impression at the periphery.

III. MIXED OR COMBINED QUANTITATIVE AND QUALITATIVE MODIFICATIONS OF ELECTRICAL IRRITABILITY.

Atypical Forms of Reaction of Degeneration (Partial R. D. of Erb).—In these cases there may be complete abolition of the power to conduct motor impulses, but the intensity of the galvanic and faradic irritability remains normal, or is slightly diminished. The farado-muscular excitability remains, but the characteristic sluggish contraction with hyper-irritability is manifested upon testing for the galvano-muscular reaction.

The farado-muscular irritability may be diminished, or the contraction may be tardy, or exhibit a staccato movement (faradic R. D., Erb). Stintzing produced this form of reaction of degeneration in the rabbit after moderate nerve-stretching. Von Ziemssen and Stintzing have also observed it in a case of rheumatic facial paralysis.

In rare instances the neuro-faradic irritability may be lost, while the neuro-galvanic irritability is maintained intact. Adamkiewicz has observed the direct contrary effect.

Partial reaction of degeneration has also been observed in cases of central lesion in which the electrical neuro-irritability had been maintained, and indeed in cases in which there was no muscular paralysis present. Von Ziemssen has observed this reaction in a case of lead-paresis, in which there was diminution but not entire loss of voluntary muscular power.

Stintzing has recently published an interesting contribution upon the reaction of degeneration, in which he has classified the forms of R. D. in four groups, as follow: 1. R. 1)., with total loss of neuro-irritability. 2. R. D., with partial loss of neuro-irritability. 3. R. D. , with sluggish faradic irritability of the nerve. 4. R. D., with prompt neuro-irritability to both currents.

Diagnostic and Prognostic Significance of Reaction of Degeneration. — The phenomena of reaction of degeneration characterize all varieties and degrees of peripheral paralysis of motion, no matter whether they are traumatic, rheumatic, neuritic, or diphtheritic in origin. In cases of this character 11. D. is such an essential part of the clinical history of the affection that, when contrasted with its absence in central or purely myopathic lesions, it was formerly believed to furnish an absolutely diagnostic sign. But more recently, as pointed out above, certain diseases of the spinal cord, especially such as are dependent upon lesions in the anterior gray columns of the cord and the nuclear region of the medulla, were also-found to be attended by the phenomena of reaction of degeneration.' Among the diseases of the spinal cord in which R. D. is found are infantile spinal paralysis (anterior poliomyelitis), lead-paralysis, and primary progressive muscular atrophy. It is also present exceptionally in amyotrophic lateral sclerosis, progressive bulbar paralysis, spinal hemorrhage and tumors, secondary amyotrophies, and diphtheritic paralyses of the trunk and extremities.

Reaction of degeneration is absent in all cerebral, hysterical, myelitic, and purely myopathic paralyses. In cases where the R. D. is limited to a definite peripheral neuro-muscular area, the probabilities are in favor of the diagnosis of a peripheral lesion. When the phenomena of R. D. are observed over a larger area, a central (spinal) origin of the paralysis is rendered probable.

The prognostic significance of R. D. is often of assistance to the physician. "Where the phenomena exhibited arc of-slight degree, the prognosis is, on the whole, favorable, but when faradic irritability is entirely lost, the galvanic irritability greatly increased, and the contractions very sluggish with the typical reversal of the normal formula of contraction, or where all electrical irritability is lost,—in these cases a favorable prognosis cannot be safely hazarded until the reappearance of the normal formula of contraction.

Diagnosis of Disturbances of Common Sensation.—Erb devised an electrode for testing the sensibility of the skin. This electrode consists of about four hundred fine, insulated wires fastened compactly in a handle. The ends of the wires are then ground off evenly, thus presenting a smooth surface with a number of contact points corresponding to the number of wires. An ingenious modification of this electrode is shown in Fig. 168. The surface of the disk, two centimetres in diameter, is subdivided by a saw into a large number of fields (250-300) and the clefts made by the saw filled out with some non-conducting material. To test the sensation, this electrode attached to the secondary coil of the induction machine is applied to the surface to be tested, and the other electrode to an indifferent point, *e.g.,* the sternum. The coils are then shoved over each other until the sensation of the current is just perceptible. This is marked as "x mm. C. D.," and then the coil is further advanced until the first sensation of pain is experienced, and the C. 1). again recorded. The first record shows the minimum sensation reaction, while the second shows the minimum painful reaction. The corresponding reaction on, the opposite side of the body is then ascertained and the results compared with each other.

Diminution of sensory irritability is present in most serious lesions of the spinal cord and peripheral nerves, and in many cerebral affections.

Fig. 1B8.—Electrode For Testing Electro-cutaneous Sensibility.

Von Ziemssen has attempted to measure the time of sensory impressions (the diminution of pain conduction) by means of the discharge of a Leyden jar. No practical results of importance have, however, as yet been obtained.

Bernhardt has tested the reaction of cutaneous sensibility and finds that it varies in different areas or "zones" of the body. He divides the surface of the body into nine zones, as follows:— 1. Tongue zone (tip of tongue, palate, tip of nose).
2. Face zone (eyelids, gums, red surface of lips, cheek). 3. Forehead zone (forehead, cutaneous surface of lips). 4. Shoulder zone (shoulder). 5. Trunk zone (sternum, nape of neck, spine, arm, forearm, buttock, occiput, front of neck). 6. Thigh zone (sacrum, thigh, dorsum of foot). 7. Hand zone (back of hand, leg, ball of fingers). 8. Patellar zone (patella). 9. Digital zone (tip of toes, palm of hand, sole of foot).
The average minimum C. D. of sensation and of pain for
these various regions is given in the following table:— *Reactions of Electromuscular Sensibility.*—Duchenne first called attention to a peculiar *sensation* in the muscle when a current of electricity is acting upon or through it. This sensation is not dependent upon the sensibility of the skin, but is quite different from and independent of it. This '-electromuscular sensibility" may be present even in cases of cutaneous anaesthesia, or where the muscles are exposed in consequence of detachment of the skin from accident. The pathological significance of this electro-muscular sensibility has not received much attention. Some clinical observations of Dr. S. Weir Mitchell are, however, interesting in this connection. He found that when the cut ends of the nerves in an amputation stump are irritated by an electric current the patient can describe the sensations of movement of certain muscles in the amputated extremity. "If we faradize the track of the nerves in or above the stump," says Dr. Mitchell, "we may cause the lost fingers and thumb to seem to be flexed or extended, and, what is most remarkable, parts of which the man is conscious, but which he has not tried to stir for years, may thus be made to appear to move to his utter amazement. In one case I thus acted on the nerves so as to cause a thumb, which for years was constantly and violently bent in on the palm, to straighten out completely. On breaking the circuit, without warning, the patient exclaimed that his thumb was cutting the palm again, and the same result was obtained by shifting the conductors so as to put the nerves out of the circuit. Injuries of Nerves, p. 360.

"In a case of amputation at the shoulder-joint, in which all consciousness of the limb had long since vanished, I suddenly faradized the brachial plexus, when the patient said at once: 'My hand is there again. It is all bent up and hurts me.' These impressions are correctly referred by the patient, so that faradization of the musrulo-spiral or the ulnar gives sensation of movement in the related parts. It is, of course, impossible that the motor nerves stimulated should convey any impression centrally, and we must therefore conclude that irritation of sensory trunks may occasion impressions of muscular motion in the sensorium."

Electro-muscular anaesthesia is found in cases of hysteria and tabes dorsalis. It is often combined with cutaneous anaesthesia and analgesia, although either may be present without the other.

Electrical Reaction Of The Organs Of Special Sense. *Eye.*—In testing the reaction of the optic nerve for purposes of diagnosis the same procedure is followed as in testing the normal reaction (page 155). Weak currents must be employed, increasing the same very gradually by means of a rheostat. The ordinary resistance coils generally furnished with the medical apparatus do not answer for this purpose. One of the more recent devices, by means of which the current can be increased or diminished by almost imperceptible gradations, must be used. (See Figs. 196 and 197.)

No very trustworthy results have yet been obtained in the use of the electric current for diagnostic purposes in pathological conditions of the visual organs. Only a modification in the intensity of the normal reaction to the electrical stimulus has been observed.

Ear.—The diagnosis of ear diseases by electricity has been pretty thoroughly worked out by some observers. It is found that in some affections the normal formula of Brenner is preserved with quantitative changes, *i.e.,* the intensity of the sensation is either increased or diminished. In other cases (especially diseases of the labyrinth) there is complete reversal of the normal formula, as in R. D. The practical application of these results is as yet insignificant. The same may be said of the diagnostic value of electricity in disorders of the olfactory and gustatory nerves.

The Electric Light As An Aid In Diagnosis.

That "seeing is believing" is an axiom especially dear to the medical and surgical practitioner. For the purpose of making an exact diagnosis, direct vision in a good light is regarded as highly important. For this reason particularly, attempts have been made for many years to render certain internal organs accessible to direct ocular inspection. It is, however, only within the last ten years that the practical ingenuity of mechanicians has furnished a set of instruments which can readily be used for diagnostic purposes, and in which the electric light is made practically available.

In the first part of this work, the physical principles governing the production of the electric light have been treated at sufficient length. It remains here merely to give an account of the various instruments used for the purpose, and the results thus far attained.

Among the medical and surgical instruments having the electric light as a basis, those most commonly used are the stomatoscope, laryngoscope, otoscope, urethroscope, cystoscope, and gastroscope. The most perfect forms of these instruments available at the present day are those constructed by Josef Leiter, the well-known surgical-instrument maker, of Vienna, although some practical modifications have recently been introduced by other manufacturers.

As the production of a sufficiently intense light to render an instrument available for the exploration of any internal cavity or organ is necessarily accompanied by the development of a degree of heat. which may render the use of the instrument impracticable if not counteracted, the instruments of Leiter are surrounded by a current of water which is kept constantly circulating and which carries off the excess of heat. In Figs. 169 and 170 the general construction of Leiter's apparatus is shown. The description is taken from an article by Dr. Roswell Park, of Buffalo:—

"i? is a hard-wood box containing three large Bunsen cells with double zinc plates exposing a large surface. They are so arranged in a hard-rubber cell, witli large bottles *of* battery fluids on either side, that by means of a rubber bulb and glass tube they can be filled or emptied by simply siphoning the fluids in and out. Simple directions enable the operator to connect one, two or three elements as desired. For ordinary endoscopic purposes, two, or even one, suffice; for galvano-cautery all three are needed. Wires from 1 and 2 on the battery box run to 1 and 2 at /?, which is the rheostat. With the pointer at *0,* the position it occupies in the cut, there is no current; as it is turned around on the index scale the resistance is diminished, until with the pointer way round the circle all resistance is out of the circuit. At 3 and 4 are the wires which run to the instrument in use, as, for instance, the laryngoscope at *L.* By a simple spring-clamp they are put on or removed in an instant.

"*S* is a metallic tubular reser.voir about one metre in height, also shown in cross-section. This is filled with four litres of

» A storage battery would be more efficient and convenient.

cool water. A heavy leaden weight or plunger (ten kilos), *bg,* is swung from the under surface of the cover by pulleys, *ro;* the cord attached to the little handle, *gr,* serves to hoist it; *ko* is a closely-fitting piston having a valve, *ve,* which allows the weight to be raised, but causes it to rest on the surface of the water, which, by its weight, is driven up through «»', its flow being checked or regulated by the stop-cock,/, at its upper end.

Fig. 1W.—Combined Battery And Hydrostatic Apparatus.

Water being thus caused to flow, passes around the rheostat and through the tube, *h,* by flexible-rubber tubes into the instrument, around the heated wire, back through the tube *k* at *m,* where it drops back into the reservoir at *tr;* and can be used over and over again. With proper adjustment the weight need not be raised oftener than once in twenty minutes, but the water must *s* be kept steadily flowing, or there is danger to the instruments. At *p* is a metal loop in which the tubes and wires may rest so that their weight is hardly noticed. At *l l* are handles by winch the whole instrument can be moved about as desired."

The urethroscope is shown in detail in Fig. 170, and in position in Fig. 171. Tho outer tube or cannula, *in,* is about the size of a catheter No. 21 F. Into this is pushed the rectangular tube, *b b,* containing the illuminating and cooling The loop of platinum wire, *c,* is seen at the lower beveled end of this part of the apparatus. In one of the water tubes is an insulated wire, the other conductor being furnished by the main body of the metal work. The cold water passes into the tube at *h,* and arrangement ifter flowing through the entire length of the apparatus, but without coming in contact with the heated wire, passes out at *i.* The funnel-shaped extremity, *7c,* is the eye-piece.

In Fig. 171 the instrument is shown in position. With it a surface of one centimetre square can be illuminated at one time. It will be readily seen how useful this apparatus may be made in the diagnosis of diseased conditions of the urethral mucous membrane.

Annals of Anatomy and Surgery, March, 1883. -The UreThroscope In PoSition.

The cystoscope is a further development of the instrument just described. It is shown complete in Fig. 172. Fig. 173 shows the cystoscope in position illuminating the interior of the bladder. Leiter has recently still further improved the cystoscope, and claims now to be able to use the electric light for purposes of interior illumination without the necessity of the

Fig. 17Z—The Cystoscope. refrigerating apparatus. This is a great advance in simplicity, and will promote the use of these instruments by reducing their cost, which is still a great drawback.

An otoscope of simpler construction has been devised by Dr. Roswell Park, which is shown in Fig. 174. Its use is practicable either in broad daylight or in a dark room.

Laryngoscopes and rhinoscopes are made upon the same principle. Fig. 175 shows the method of using the former.

There are many modifications of these instruments now obtainable. A very simple and cheap one, which may be used as a stomatoscope and pharyngoscope, is that shown in Fig. 176. The glow-lamp is affixed to the end of a tongue-depressor.

The highest development of the electrical illumination of internal cavities has been reached in the gastroscope, which is the result of the collaboration of Professor Mikulicz and Mr. Leiter. The instrument is shown in position in the stomach in Fig. 177. Its method of use is described by Dr. Park as follows:—

"As preparation for the use of the gastroscope, it is necessary that the patient shall have gone for some hours without eating. Half an hour previous to its use a hypodermic dose of morphia—say, one-third grain—should be administered. Just prior to the examination the stomach should be washed out. The patient is then laid upon the left side on a table having a head-support, which shall keep the neck in its axial position. A small receptacle is placed under the mouth to catch the saliva which cannot be swallowed. The head is then thrown well back, and the instrument, which has previously been lubricated with vaseline or glycerine, is guided by the finger of the left hand and passed downward with a gentle sweep. Previous practice on the cadaver with a hard-rubber sound of the same dimensions and flexure as the gastroscope will easily teach the necessary manipulations. The instrument being in place, the stomach is inflated to the desired extent, but not sufficient to distress the patient. The pointer on the rheostat being turned slowly, the metal blind is drawn and the observer has the field before him."

With reference to the value of these various devices, Dr. Park, who is entitled to speak from experience, says: "I feel justified in saying that, in expert hands and with an expert's eye at the eye-piece, the instrument may and ought to play a *role* in diagnosis which has never heen filled before. It deserves a careful study of itself and an extended trial; until it has had both, its merits should not be disregarded."

Fig. 170—Tongue-iiepresbor, With Fig. 177.—The Uastuoscope In Position. Electric Light.

THE TELEPHONE AS AN AID TO DIAGNOSIS.

Dr. Boudet, of Paris, has devised a number of instruments in which the telephone and microphone are availed of as aids to diagnosis. These instruments arc the sphygmophone, sphygmophonic transmitter, and myophone. By means of the latter the inventor has been enabled to make a differential diagnosis between various paretic conditions of muscles. Hughes' sonometer is an electrical apparatus to determine the degree of deafness. The instrument is of limited applicability.

Annals of Anatomy and Surgery, March, 1883.

The induction balance and telephonic probe, invented by A. Graham Bell, for the purpose of detecting metallic bodies of various sorts—*e.g.*, bullets—in the deeper tissues, have been used several times, but with only moderate success.

ELECTRO-THERMOMETRY.

Dr. F. Arnheim has recently devised an electrical thermoscopc for the purpose of determining the radiation of the bodyheat. The apparatus consists of a delicate thermopile, containing forty pairs of iron and German-silver wires arranged in series, and a delicate galvanometer. The apparatus is doubtless valuable for physiological researches, but in its present state is of little use for the purposes of the clinician.

ELECTROLYTIC ANALYSTS.

For the purpose of detecting minute quantities of any metal in the secretions or tissues of the body electrolysis mav be employed. A convenient apparatus for this purpose has lately been described by Professor Wolff.

The decomposing part of the apparatus is a glass cylindrical cell, J, having a globular extension on top, an outlet tube,/, at one side, and an inlet or receiving tube at the other side, 7t, below; the positive electrode is made of strong platinum wire in form of a spiral, which is resting close against the inner wall of the cylinder, with its lower end sealed in and reaching outside to a binding-screw, n, at the support; the negative electrode is also spiral-shaped, but made of thin iron wire, which has been copper-and afterward silver-plated; it is supported centrally in the interior of the cylinder, A, by a cork at the neck of the latter, and receives the current by a small clamp on a sliding-rod Notes on New Remedies, from Fischer's Zeitschrift f. Augewandte C'hcmie. and a binding-screw, z, at its base, to connect with the zinc pole of the battery.

The liquid to be analyzed, supposing it to contain mercury, after being weighed, then acidulated with 3 to 4 per cent, of sulphuric acid, is contained in a funnel-shaped reservoir, which is connected by a rubber pipe with 7c, by which it enters into the decomposing cell, the influx of the liquid being regulated by a Bunsen screw-clamp, so that one drop in about five seconds enters at h and is discharged at /, and the electric current passing the electrodes in the same direction. In the same measure as the liquid is passing upward, the mercury is precipi tated on the silver-plated cathode. After the liquid has passed through the cell, the rest left in the latter is discharged from it by a current of pure water, until the generation of gas at the electrodes has entirely ceased. The negative spiral is then removed from the cell, washed carefully with water, then with alcohol, and last with ether, and, perfectly dry, is separated from the wire end, and transferred to a glass tube of six millimetres diameter, open at the lower end, and open and drawn out to a narrow tube on top; the lower open end of this tube is then sealed as in Fig. 179, d, the tube then carefully heated over a gas or alcohol flame to a red heat from the closed end, where the spiral is placed upward, and under continuous revolving, until all the mercury precipitated on the spiral has been volatilized, and appears as a sublimate at the narrow part of the tube. In cases where the quantity of mercury, contained in a liquid, and now received as a sublimate, is excessively small, the latter may be detected by subjecting it to well-known chemical tests.

The sensibility of this method of detecting mercury is quite extraordinary; quantities of to milligramme of the metal in one hundred cubic centimetres of liquid give by its correct application the most distinct reactions, and its value for physiological analysis is therefore an acknowledged one.

The intensity of the current necessary for the electrolytic separation of the mercury is one of 100 to 150 milliamperes, equal to a current necessary to produce one and two-tenths to one and five-tenths cubic centimetres oxyhydrogen gas in one minute. The copper plating of the negative spiral is done by dipping the same for a few minutes in diluted sulphuric acid one to five parts, exposing it for one minute to the action of the negative pole of a copper-zinc battery in a bath of a concentrated solution of cupric sulphate, acidulated with sulphuric acid; the positive electrode being a spiral of strong copper wire. The silver plating is then performed in a similar manner in four to five minutes, with a positive spiral of platinum wire, in a silver solution consisting of five grammes argentic nitrate, twenty-five grammes potassic cyanide, in two hundred and fifty cubic centimetres water, with an intensity of current of 100 milliamperes.

If the decomposing cell *A,* herein described, is used for the electrolytic analysis of other metals than mercury, as, for instance, for copper, silver, etc. , the negative spiral used must be also of platinum, and in this case the precipitated metal adhering to the spiral may for identical reaction be washed into a test-tube, and then dissolved by adding a small quantity of nitric acid.

CHAPTER III.

Methods Of Applying The Electric Current For Therapeutic

Purposes. *Instruments and Appliances.*—Electricity is employed for therapeutic purposes in the form of the constant or galvanic current, or *galvanism,* the induced or faradic current, or *faro dism,* and static or frictional electricity, or *franklinism.* Each of these varieties of electricity requires different apparatus for its administration, with which the practitioner must be familiar before he can employ this agent rationally.

Appliances for Using the Constant Current—Batteries.— The construction and action of galvanic batteries have been described in detail in the first part of this work, to which the reader is referred. In this chapter it remains to mention the arrangements for various medical and surgical purposes.

Medical batteries are simply modifications or combinations of the different elements or cells, of which illustrations are given in Chapter III, Part L The principles and laws governing the arrangement of elements for the development of certain physical phenomena are likewise applicable in the construction of batteries for medical and surgical use. Thus, in one case a battery is desired which shall overcome great resistance. Here we need high electro-motive force, and in order to secure this we arrange the cells in series. In another case we have slight resistance to overcome, but desire a large current. In this instance we connect the cells "for quantity " or in multiple arc. These terms have been fully explained on pages 104 and 105.

Galvanic batteries for medical purposes may naturally be divided into two classes,—stationary and portable.

Stationary Batteries.—A stationary or office battery should possess the following desiderata: It should give a steady current of the quality needed, should not give off acrid fumes, be easily kept clean, require little attention, and keep in good working order for a considerable time. Among the batteries in use, the Leclanche, or one of its modifications, fulfills most of these desiderata. There are, however, other batteries which are useful, and which may for a particular class of work give better results. Among these may be mentioned the Siemens-IIalske cell, which is a modification of the Daniell. It has, however, a very high internal resistance, and where hvrge currents are required, as in some classes of gynaecological work, it fails to meet the demands made upon it. A further objection to its use is the tendency of the salts to "creep," and cause incrustation of the sides of the jars. The cell is, however, very constant, and requires little attention.

Storage batteries arc now made which answer the demands of an office battery almost to perfection. When their management is thoroughly understood, and the current they furnish regulated by a proper rheostat, they give little trouble and save much annoyance. They may either be charged at an electriclight station, by an incandescent-light wire, or by a few cells of gravity battery..

Many instrument-makers have constructed cabinets to contain the batteries and other appliances for office use. The cells used in these cabinets are usually some form of Leclanche element. Much ingenuity has been expended in securing convenience of arrangement as well as elegance of finish in these cabinets. Waite & Bartlett, of New York, Otto Flemming, of Philadelphia, and the Mcintosh Galvanic and Faradic Battery Company, of Chicago, make cabinet batteries with which all sorts of medical electrical work except galvano-causty can be performed. The accompanying illustration shows the office cabinet, as made by Waite & Bartlett. The cells, as shown, are contained in the cupboard, which forms the base of the piece of furniture. In the upper portion are a handy arrangement for switching into action the cells, automatic galvanic interrupter, or rheotome, commutator, metallic and water rheostats, an excellent faradic apparatus, and a milliamperemeter for measuring the strength of the current. There are also drawers and spaces for putting away electrodes and appliances.

The office cabinet of Otto Flemming is also conveniently arranged and of excellent workmanship.

Fig. 182.—Massey's Movable Table.

An arrangement to take the place of office cabinets, where economy of space in the room is an object, is known among instrument-makers as a wall cabinet. Many useful forms of this apparatus are made, the most complete and handy being shown in the cut (Fig. 181). The cells may be put in a closet, cellar, or distant room and connected with the switch-board by insulated wires. The wall cabinet is well adapted for hospitals and dispensaries, as it furnishes the current in convenient arrangement, without occupying much space in the operating room.

A convenient movable table for hospital work has been designed by Dr. G. Betton Massey. It is shown in Fig. 182.

Where the electrical bath is used, some convenient method of switching the currents off and on and reversing currents is

Fig. 183.—Fakadic-batu Apparatus. often desired. The manufacturers have supplied this in an exceedingly useful switch-board, one of which is illustrated in Fig. 183. This is made by the Mcintosh Galvanic and Faradic Battery Company, of Chicago.

Portable Batteries.—The frequent necessity of applying electricity at the patient's residence has stimulated instrument makers to an active rivalry in making portable galvanic batteries. In addition to the desiderata, already mentioned, which should be possessed by a stationary battery, the portable battery makes another demand, namely, that it should *be* portable. This at once excludes those elements whose greatest excellence is their steadiness of action, namely, the Leclanche and the various sulphate of copper cells. Their size and weight preclude their use as portable batteries. The storage battery has not yet been sufficiently developed in this direction to furnish a sufficiently high electro-motive force consistent with portability.

Hence, it also must be excluded from consideration in this connection. We are restricted, therefore, in making a choice of cell for a portable battery to the bichromate cell, the bisulphate of mercury cell, and the chloride of silver cell. All of these have been used in constructing batteries, of which the following figures show useful designs.

Bichromate Batteries.—The batteries shown in Figs. 184, 185, and 186 are convenient and efficient in action, as tested by the writer personally. The cells are of hard rubber or glass, and when the battery is not in use the elements are removed from the solution by lowering the tray, as in the Flemming and Waite & Bartlett batteries, or by placing them in empty com

Fig. 183.—Flemming's Thirty-cell Galvanic Battery. partments, as in the Mcintosh instrument. To prevent spilling of the fund while carrying the Flemming, or Waite & Bartlett battery, a padded board, called a hydrostat, is shoved in between the tops of the cells and the ends of the zinc-carbon elements, and, by means of screws the board is brought firmly against the tops of the cells, thus effectually sealing them.

Solution of bisulphate of mercury may be used in these batteries instead of the acid solution of potassium bichromate, but it does not give a sufficiently strong current for many purposes.

The disadvantages of these forms of batteries are the following: The fluid soon becomes weak and requires to be changed; the cells become leaky, and, where hard-rubber cells are used, a complete new tray or set is required when only one cell is

Fig. 187.—Barrett Chloride Of Silver Hatteey. defective. This becomes a source of expense. Glass cells, especially where toughened glass is used, are more durable. Unless great care is taken in screwing up the hydrostat the fluid may spill and corrode any metal points it reaches. This may give rise to defective contacts and so interfere with the efficiency of the apparatus.

In spite, however, of these shortcomings the bichromate batteries remain, at present, our best type of portable batteries, being moderate in price, furnishing a strong1 current, and, where intelligently and carefully handled, not being very liable to get out of order.

Chloride of Silver Batteries.—For neatness, portability, and convenience of arrangement the chloride of silver "dry" battery shown in Fig. 187 leaves little to be desired. It is made by the John A. Barrett Battery Company, of Baltimore, and the designer claims to have secured a constant, uniform, and durable current. Previous experiences with other forms of this battery, *e.g.,* Gaiffe's, have, however, not proven satisfactory. The first expense is considerable, and the life of the cell is too short. When the chloride of silver is reduced to metallic silver, the usefulness of the battery is at an end until the elements are replaced by others. The company making the battery shown above offer to replace worn-out cells with new ones at a small cost. Most of these portable galvanic batteries are also furnished with a faradic apparatus, but the physician should keep these two instruments separate. Neither the portability nor efficiency of the apparatus is increased by a "combination" of two different instruments in the same case.

Faradic Batteries.—Faradic batteries are usually made in portable form. Unfortunately, there is, at present, no standard in use among American manufacturers. Many of the faradic machines in the market are very imperfectly constructed. The best makers have adopted the Du Bois-Reymond coil as a model, but in all except the more expensive instruments little care is taken to make a good, trustworthy apparatus. The scale to indicate the coil distance, when furnished at all, is often of no value whatever as an indication of the current strength.

An excellent Du Bois-Rcymond coil is made by Flemming. This has a double scale, the zero upon which indicates the zero of current, whether the primary or secondary current is used. The outer coil is propelled by means of a screw, enabling the practitioner to increase or diminish the current in the most gradual manner. This instrument, which lacks the element of portability, is usually set in action with a Grenet cell. This apparatus is shown in Fig. 188.

The above illustration (Fig. 189) shows an exceedingly convenient and handy faradic battery, in which the chloride of silver cell is the motive agent. It seems to work well, and possesses the advantage of portability and ease of management in a very high degree. It is guaranteed to run without diminution of current for one hundred hours. For accurate observations, however, the scale showing the coil distance—the only method now available for approximately measuring the current of a faradic machine—should be more carefully made than heretofore.

Fig. 190.—Engeljiakn's Faeadic Batteey, With Three Coils.

Two or three years ago Dr. George J. Engelmann, of St. Louis, devised a faradic apparatus, shown in Fig. 190, which appears to have many advantages over the ordinary batteries sold for physicians' use. This battery is provided with three coils of different-sized wires, and different resistances, which are marked upon the coils. These coils are termed, respectively, coarse, fine, and medium. According to Dr. Engelmann, the coarse coil should be used for muscular contractions, and to produce contraction of the uterus when in a condition of subinvolution, the fine coil to relieve the pain in cellulitis, and the medium to produce muscular contractions when the parts are too sensitive to permit the use of the coarse coil. This battery was primarily designed for use in gynaecological cases; but every practitioner conversant with the effects of faradic electricity will see indications for the use of the different coils. It is earnestly to be desired that careful observations should be made with this apparatus.

A faradta battery, which can be readily carried in the coatpocket, is made by (iaiife, of Paris, and by several American

Fig. 191.—Uaiffe's Faradic Poceet Battery. firms. The galvanic current is furnished by two small carbon trays, representing the carbon element, and two flat, square blocks of zinc for the positive element. The exciting fluid is solution of mercury bisulphate. A current of considerable intensity can be obtained from this little instrument, and it may often be employed to advantage.

ACCESSORY APPARATUS.

Current Selector.—Every battery should be so arranged that any one cell, or any number of cells can be thrown into circuit when wanted. In many of the stationary apparatuses now before the profession the current selector or switch is defective in this particular, there being no way of picking out cells in the series, unless the first cells are also included. Most recent devices have this defect corrected. Purchasers of stationary electrical apparatus should insist upon being furnished with the form of switch known as the "Universal" Current Selector, hy means of which any individual cell, or number of cells in the series, may be switched into circuit.

Commutator, or Pole Changer.—For the purpose of rapid reversal of the direction of the current (voltaic alternation), nearly all galvanic batteries have a simple switch, called a commutator, attached. By means of this arrangement the direction of the current, or, what is the same thing, the relative positions of the poles, can be changed without removing the

Fig. 192.—Lewis' Pedal Commutator
Fig. 193.—Flemming's Automatic

And Rheotome. Kueotome. electrodes from the body. It is essential that the springs by which the contacts are made in the commutator shall work stiffly, otherwise the contact is liable to be defective.

Dr. Morris J. Lewis, of Philadelphia, has devised an ingenious commutator and circuit-breaker, to be operated with the feet (Fig. 192). The posts *P* and *N* are connected with the positive and negative poles, respectively, of the battery. The electrodes are connected with the binding-posts *A* and *B*. The circuit is made and broken with the pedal at the side of the instrument. By pressing on the button *A* with the other foot, the electrode connected with the binding-post *A* becomes positive; by pressing on the button *B,* the electrode running to *B* becomes positive.

Current Interrupter, or Rheotome.— Where it is desired to interrupt the galvanic current at regular intervals, an automatic rheotome, or contact-breaker, is necessary. In some instruments the interruptions are made by clock-work, which can be set fast or slow, as in the one shown in Fig. 193. The figures above the buttons indicate the number of interruptions per second. In other forms of the instrument the interruptions are produced by the vibration of the armature of a small electro-magnet. The amplitude of the vibration determines the intervals between the interruptions. Some faradic machines have attachments for slow interruptions of the induced current, which are often advantageous in diagnosis. *Milliamperemeter.* — The proper "dosage" of electricity has only recently attracted much attention on the part of the profession. The former practice, which, indeed, still prevails to a very great extent, has been to state the strength of current in the number of cells used. The reader who has carefully studied the first part of this work need not be told that this method of estimating the strength of current used is entirely fallacious. Not only do different cells vary in the electro-motive force and current furnished, but the same cells differ at different times, owing to conditions fully set forth in a previous section. The size and character of the electrodes used, the resistance of the portion of the body operated upon, and the manner in which the electrodes are applied, all control, to a greater or less degree, the available strength of current at the point of application. Hence, in order to determine exactly how much current is traversing the tissues, and, probably, doing certain work there in modifying nutrition, etc. , a means is desirable by which we can measure the current, to find out, as it may be expressed, the *dose* of electricity which we are administering to the patient. Such an apparatus is at our command in the so-called absolute galvanometer or milliamperemeter, shown on the following page.

The milliampere has been adopted by common consent among therapeutists as the electro-therapeutic unit, and it has become customary to record the strength of the galvanic current used in any case in milliamperes (Ma). While the use of this instrument has only very recently become general, and no fixed rules as to the measured current strength to be used in all dis

FIg. 194.— MILLIaMPEREMETER. eases have yet been established, certain important results have already been obtained to which reference will be made in the next chapter. Electrolytic operations, especially, have yielded much more definite results since the measuring of the current used has been more regularly practiced.

It is therefore most earnestly urged upon the practitioner who uses the galvanic current that the milliamperemeter should be a constant accessory to the battery in the application of electro-therapy and diagnosis. The proper construction of this instrument has been described in the first part of this work.

In all stationary batteries now made by the instrument-makers it is an essential part of the outfit. It should, in addition, be used also in measuring the current when a portable battery is used. Fig. 195 shows the instrument connected in circuit with a portable battery.

Rheostat, or Current Controller.—In the practical application of electricity it is often desirable to use a less strength of current than is furnished by a single cell, or to increase or diminish the current more gradually than can be done by the addition or dropping out of circuit single cells-by means of the current selector. For this purpose a carefully graduated rheostat should be used. The rheostats usually furnished with galvanic batteries are in the form of resistance coils, each of which when switched into the circuit introduces a certain definite resistance depending upon the length, thickness, and kind of wire used. (See "Resistance," Part I.) But these forms of rheostat are not suitable for medical purposes, where an instrument is required that will gradually—almost imperceptibly—vary the current strength instead of increasing or diminishing it *per salt um,* as happens in the older form of resistance coils.

An excellent resistance instrument is the water rheostat (Fig. 196), which permits a very gradual increase or decrease in the current. It is, however, more suitable for interposition in a faradic than in a galvanic circuit, for when the latter current passes through the water electrolysis of the liquid immediately begins, which soon itself adds to the resistance by coating one of the contact points with hydrogen gas.

Fig. 19-). — Method Of Con.vecting Mli.i.iamperemetek To Portable Battery.

A more recent form of the water rheostat is the "Baily Current Regulator" (Fig. 197), manufactured by the Law Battery Company, of New York. The place of the rod of metal in the ordinary water rheostat is taken in this instrument by four carbon plates tapering to a point. The current can be very gradually increased or decreased with this rheostat. Among other forms highly recommended are the graphite rheostat of Dr. Gartner, of Vienna, and a modification of this instrument by Dr. G. Betton Masscy, and figured in his book.

Fig. 196.—Water Rheostat.
Fig. 107.—Daily Current Regulator.

Electrodes, on Rheophores.—Electrodes are instruments through which electricity is applied to the body. They vary in size and shape with the special purpose for which they are used.
Electricity In the Diseases of Women. Philadelphia: F. A. Davis. 1888.

Those most frequently used are the ordinary flat electrodes, one and one-half inches in diameter, and covered with sponge, or absorbent cotton, as suggested by Dr. G. Betton Massey. The absorbent-cotton covering is much neater and cleaner than the sponge, and should come into general use. A new cover is used for each sitting. This electrode is only slightly larger than the "normal electrode" of Erb, and may be used ordinarily as a testing electrode in electro-diagnosis. The surface of all electrodes should be of metal, nickel-plated, or of carbon. For the galvanic current the carbon electrodes are better, as they are not corroded by the electrolytic action when a saline solution is used to moisten them. The cut (Fig. 198) shows a number of the electrodes used by Erb. The smaller ones are used for fine nerve-branches and small muscles, while the larger ones are used for determining the quantitative reaction of various muscles. The "indifferent" electrode of Erb has a surface of fifty square centimetres, is oblong in shape, with a slightly concave surface, and well padded with cotton. Its size is about five by ten centimetres (two by four inches). This electrode is useful in stimulating large muscles to contraction and in applying electricity to the chest, ahdomen, and thighs; where large surfaces are to be covered at a time, still larger electrodes are used by Erb, von Ziemssen, and others.

For the purpose of stimulating the sensation of the skin, or of producing reflex muscular contraction by irritation of the skin, the electric brush or scourge is used (Fig. 199).

Fig. 199.—Electric Brush.

In order to reduce the expense of an electrical outfit and to economize space, instrument-makers usually furnish a common or "universal" handle, to which all the various electrodes may be attached. Some of these handles are plain, others are provided with a key for interrupting the current. Examples of each are here shown (Figs. 200 and 201).

Some makers have introduced various complicated arrangements in the handles of electrodes. Among these are commutator handles and rheostat handles. All these accessories are, however, better introduced in some other portion of the circuit.

Fig. 207.—Skin Excttator. (Barrett.)
Fig. 208.—Skin Excitator. (Mcintosh.)

For convenience of manipulation and to secure accurate and firm adaptation of the contacts to the skin so-called "fixation electrodes" are used (Fig. 202). Those shown in the cut may be used for the neck, thigh, leg, or arm. The preceding page shows a number of special electrodes adapted for various purposes.

Fig. 203 is a flexible electrode for the application of the current to the head, or to painful surfaces, such as inflamed joints. Fig. 204, a metallic foot-plate, which can be covered with a towel moistened with a warm saline solution, thus obviating the necessity of using a sponge-covered electrode, which soon becomes dirty. Fig. 205 is an electrode with a long stem, for use along the spine, avoiding the necessity of removing the clothing. Fig. 206 is a massage electrode, which is very useful in cases of chronic inflammation of the joints and chronic inflammatory infiltrations. Figs. 207 and 208 are electrodes for producing faradic excitation of the skin in anaesthesia, or where it is desired to affect deep-seated organs by reflex action.

Other electrodes for special uses will be described in the appropriate sections in the chapter on Electro-Therapeutics.

ELECTRO-CAUTERY APPARATUS.

Batteries.—The elements of a galvano-cautery batter)' should have large surface, and the battery should have small internal resistance. The electro-motive force should be sufficient to readily overcome all the resistance of the circuit, and the current large enough to produce and maintain a sufficiently high degree of heat in the cautery points. The battery should not polarize quickly, or, in the event of this being unavoidable, should be supplied with an arrangement for rapid depolarization.

Cautery batteries should also be portable, as many operations require to be done at the patient's home. It is essential, however, that efficiency of action shall not be sacrificed to portability. In hospitals or offices, where a cautery is frequently required, a stationary battery placed in a cellar or closet, and connected with a switch-board in the operating-room, will give more satisfaction than a portable battery, because the plates and cells can be made larger. Fig. 209 shows such a stationary battery, modeled after that of Brnns. It is extremely convenient for office and hospital work. At the present day most cautery batteries are made with zinccarbon elements, and use the acid solution of potassium bichromate as the exciting fluid.

The rapid action going on in the cell causes the evolution of a large quantity of hydrogen gas, which produces polarization of the carbon plate unless it is displaced by agitating the liquid. This is done in some batteries by shaking the plates by means

Fig. 209—Mcintosii's Stationary Cal'tery Battery.

Fig. 210.—Top Of Fiffaed Battery, ShowIng Connections For Series Ami Quantity. of a treadle, in others by forcing a current of air through the fluid with a rubber bulb, or by giving the plates, which are hung on pivots, a rocking motion with the hand. One of the most convenient forms of portable cautery battery is that devised by Dr. Henry G. Piftard, of New York, and shown in Fig. 210. Storage batteries give excellent satisfaction as cautery batteries. Tbey can be charged by attaching them to a series of gravity cells (ten or twelve are sufficient), and when the battery is wanted for use it can be detached from the charging cells and carried wherever needed. When the electrodes are attached,' and the rate of discharge regulated by a rheostat, the instrument is ready for use. In Fig. 211 a storage battery for this purpose is shown. It contains three cells, and furnishes a current powerful enough for all cautery requirements.

Dynamo Machines.—Several European surgeons have used a small Gramme machine as the source of the energy required to heat cautery electrodes. Where steam, water-power, a gasengine, or an electro-motor can be obtained, a dynamo machine furnishes the ideal source of electrical energy for the physician. A compound machine of, say, a half horse-power will, so long as it is kept rotating at the proper rate of speed, furnish (1) a current of low electro-motive force and large "quantity," suitable for electro-cautery operations; (2) a current of high electro-motive force and small "quantity," suitable for electrolytic work and the general purposes of the medical electrician, and (3) a current by which an induction coil can be worked so as to give a faradic current. Naturally, this is only practicable for stationary outfits. For a portable apparatus the physician is still limited to the ordinary and storage batteries. The Mcintosh Battery

Fig. 212.—The Mcintosh Medicai, Dynamg..

Company, of Chicago, makes a dynamo machine, called "The Medical Dynamo," which seems to meet the requirements of the physician. In addition to furnishing the required current for cautery work, it will at the same time give a lighting-power sufficient for rhinoscopic or laryngoscopic work. The advantage of this combination must be readily evident. This machine is shown in Fig. 212.

Electrodes for Galvano-cautery.—The cautery electrodes consist of knives (flattened loops of platinum wire), fine and broad points, and loops. The conducting wires are of copper, a good conductor, while the burning-points consist of loops of platinum wire, which, offering more resistance to the current, is heated, while the copper wire is not at all or only slightly heated by the current. On reference to pages 43-45, the reader will find the reasons for this given more in detail.

The practical use of the galvano-cautery requires a careful study of the relations between electro-motive force, resistance,

Fig. 213.— Various-shaped Burners Ash Combinationu Handles. and current; in other words, an understanding of Ohm's law. For example, Jhe short loop of flattened wire constituting a cautery knife offers little resistance to the passage of the current, and consequently requires only a low electro-motive force, probably an electro-motive force of not over two volts, which would be furnished by a single cell of a good storage battery or by two cells of any good cautery battery. If. on the other hand, a loop of wire eight or ten inches long is to be heated, the resistance is very much increased, and a higher voltage (electro-motive force) would be requisite to overcome it, and to allow the current to produce the heating effect. It will be clear, then, at once to the reader that the mere possession of a cautery outfit will not insure success in any operation undertaken, unless the possessor has the requisite knowledge to use it properly.

Cautery electrodes consist of two parts, the cautery proper and the holder or handle. Most outfits are now furnished with what is known as a "Universal" handle, to which most of the cautery points can be attached. Fig. 213 shows such a combination handle, with ratchet-wheel to shorten the wire loop as it cuts, or rather burns, its way through the tissues. Immediately below are given illustrations of a large variety of burners, knives, points, and loops.

Fig. 214.—Laroe Cautery Handle.

Where large masses are to be removed, as in amputation of the cervix uteri, a handle with an ecraseur screw is used to shorten the wire, which passes through two conducting tubes. Fig. 214 illustrates this large handle.

OTHER ELECTRICAL INSTRU-

MENTS FOR SURGICAL PURPOSES.

For the rapid and accurate trephining and sawing of bones, and burring or rimming out exostoses, various instruments, in which electricity is used as the motive power, have been devised by surgeons and dentists. It would take up too much space to describe these in detail in this work. Attention may, however, be directed to the ingenious and elaborate development of the electro-motor in surgery, made by Dr. M. J. Roberts, of New York, in his electric osteotome.

International Journal of Surgery and Antiseptics, January, 1888.

INSTRUMENTS FOR APPLYING STATIC ELECTRICITY.

The principles of static induction and the construction of static machines have been explained in sufficient detail in the first part of this work (pages 28-27). It remains necessary to show here the methods of application of static electricity or franklin ism in the treatment of disease.

It is a matter of some interest that, while the first systematic applications of electricity for the treatment of disease were of the static or franklinic variety, this passed out of use almost altogether after the discovery of the voltaic pile, the magneto-electriq machine, and the induction coil. Within a few years past, however, improvements in the static machine have again directed attention to this form of electricity, and at the present time it is being largely employed as a therapeutic agent. Benedikt, Stein, and Lewandowski, in Germany, and A. L. Ranney, in the United States, are at present the most enthusiastic cultivators of this special field of electro-therapy.

The Static Machine.—Most of the static machines at present in use are modifications of the "influence machines" of Holtz (pages 26 and 27, Part I) and Toepler. Messrs. Queen & Co., of Philadelphia; Waite & Bartlett, of New York; and the Mcintosh Battery Company, of Chicago, make static machines that give a constant discharge of high electro-motive force.

By the use of a gas-engine or an electro-motor run by a storage battery, the presence of an assistant to turn the crank can be dispensed with. The necessary accessories in using static electricity arc, in addition to the influence machine (Fig. 215), an insulated platform and stool, a set of electrodes, Leyden jars, chains, hooks, and rods.

Prof. A. L. Ranney, who has devoted much study to this subject, gives these directions for the care of the static machine: "The machine should be placed in a perfectly dry room, and, if possible, in a position to allow the sun's rays to fall directly upon the plates. The metal parts should be rubbed briskly every morning with dry chamois-skin or silk. They should be Annual of the Universal Medical Sciences, 1888, voL v, p. 75, Fig. 215.—Ranney's Improved Holtz Induction Machine. occasionally repolished with emery paper. The bearings should be occasionally oiled and the leather belt tightened. During the summer fresh chloride of calcium should be kept within the case to absorb moisture."

Part III.
The Applications Of Electricity
IN THE
Treatment Of Disease.
CHAPTER I.
General Therapeutic Effects Of Electricity And Methods
Of Application.

Electricity is employed in medicine and surgery for a variety of purposes and in different ways. At one time its use is to stimulate nutrition; at another, to excite muscular contraction by its irritant or exciting effects acting either directly on the muscular fibre or indirectly through the nerve-supply of the muscle. Again, tlic current is used to modify the blood-supply of a part; here to relieve pain, there to exalt sensation; now to destroy tissue by the slow process of electrolysis, then to remove a part by the rapidly-acting galvano-cautery; and, finally, to furnish light and a medium of sound-transmission for diagnostic purposes.

All of these various applications and the methods by which they are used require detailed description and explanation.

Eor many years, Duchcnne, in France, and 11. Remak, in Germany, led two great opposing schools of electro-therapeutics. The French school, under the leadership of their great master to whom the electro-therapeutic art is under so many obligations, attributed nearly all the good effects of electricity to the induced or faradic current; while the German school, following Itemak, as exclusively pinned their faith to the constant or galvanic current. More recently, however, under the teaching of such eminent clinical observers as von Ziemssen, Erb, Benedikt, E. Remak, and others, in Germany; Onimus, Legros, Charcot, and Apostoli, in France; Althaus, De AVatteville, and Russell Reynolds, in England, and especially the late Dr. George M. Beard and his collaborator, Dr. A. D. Rockwell, in this country, it has been accepted that both currents have their appropriate indications, and that in some cases it is profitable to combine them for contemporaneous use, or to employ them in succession or alternately at the same sitting.

Much has been written of the different effects of the socalled "ascending" and "descending" currents, and of the different poles, upon the seat (or supposed seat) of the disease. It may be asserted, however, that at present our knowledge is not sufficiently definite to indicate that the *direction* of the current (if, indeed, we may properly speak of direction of current) has any especial influence. Electro-therapeutists are by no means agreed that the direction in which the current passes through diseased tissue is of any particular importance to the end aimed at, *i.e.,* the cure of the morbid condition. Since the physiological and therapeutical researches of Brenner and von Ziemssen, however, we are justified in attributing some importance to the particular pole used. This presupposes a correct appreciation of the objects had in view in the application of the current and a knowledge of electro-physics and electro-physiology. The physician should learn, even before he has purchased a battery and electrical outfit, that an agent so powerful for good, if properly, rationally, and intelligently used, is no less potent for harm if ignorantly or improperly employed.

Galvanism.—The galvanic current is used in medicine for its general and local effects. Its methods of application are these:— 1. General galvanization. 2. Central galvanization. 3. The galvanic bath. 4. Local galvanization. *General Galvanization.*—This consists in the use of a large metal plate, covered with a sponge or towel moistened with warm salt water, as cathode. The patient places his feet upon this plate, or he may sit upon it, the feet or buttocks being, of course, uncovered. The anode is a large sponge electrode, or the operator may use his hand instead, placing himself in the circuit. Having regulated by means of the current' selector, or rheostat, the strength of the current, which the operator should test on his own person, the patient is placed in the desired position (the sitting posture is most convenient), and the foot or buttock electrode connected with the negative pole of the battery. The sponge anode or the electrical band (well moistened) is then applied to the body in regular order, beginning with the head (where very weak currents should be used), over the face and neck, the upper extremities, the trunk, thighs, and along the spine. The current should never be strong enough to excite violent muscular contraction or give rise to severe pain.

General galvanization can be employed in connection with local galvanization in various neurotic or functional disorders of certain organs.

Central Galvanization.—Under this name Dr. Beard described a modified procedure, which consists in placing one large electrode (cathode) over the epigastrium, and the anode, in the same manner as in general galvanization, over the head, neck, upper extremities, trunk, and along the spine.

Sittings for the application of general and central galvanization may last five to fifteen minutes. If unpleasant effects or aggravation of the symptoms follow the employment of these methods, the current used may have been too strong, or the procedure unsuitable to the case.

The conditions especially suitable for treatment by general and central galvanization are the general functional neuroses,— neurasthenia, hysteria, hypochondria, headaches of various kinds, psychoses, chorea, and general depression of the vital powers.

Electric Bath.— The electric bath, after remaining in the exclusive possession of ignorant quacks and charlatans for many years, has recently been subjected to thorough study by scientific electro-therapeutists, chief among whom are Stein, Eulenburg, and Lehr. The technique of the electric bath has been particularly developed by the two last-named observers, who have also endeavored to more definitely establish its physiological effects and therapeutic applications. Although some encouraging results have been obtained, the indications for this method of applying electricity still lack precision. Either the constant or faradic current may be employed in the electric bath.

The methods of using the bath are various. We speak of unipolar and bipolar, or multipolar general electric baths, and of local electric baths. The arrangements for these are, briefly, as follow:—

Unipolar Bath.—The bath-tub itself, with its contained water, constitutes one electrode, while the other consists of a metal rod fixed at a convenient height above the bath-tub. The circuit is made and broken by grasping and letting go this rod, with the hands. If the bath-tub itself is of non-conducting material, metal terminals are inserted in the walls of the tub and connected with the conducting cords. There may be one or many of these points of contact.

The body of the patient is prevented from touching the metal sides and bottom of the tub, or the electrodes, by a light lattice-work of wood.

Bipolar Bath.—In the bipolar or multipolar bath the current enters at one side of the tub and passes out at the other through flat electrodes,—usually copper plates of large size, called "shovel electrodes" from their general shape.

According to Eulenburg, the unipolar bath answers all purposes for which the electric bath can be necessary, although Lehr states that the bipolar bath is more agreeable and convenient. The electric bath can be employed in the sick-room by using one of the portable rubber or canvas bath-tubs, and passing the current through the water by means of two or more large plate electrodes.

The indications for electric baths are, general functional neuroses, lowered nutrition, chronic gout and rheumatism, multiple neuralgias, tremor, neurotic skin affections (pemphigus and dermatitis herpetiformis), cerebral and spinal irritation, neurasthenia, hypochondria, etc. In hysteria, hystero-epilepsy, and heart affections this form of general electrization is contraindicated.

Localized Galvanization.—The study of the local effects of galvanism has been much advanced by the laborious investigations of R. Remak, Brenner, von Ziemssen, Erb, and others. Many of the results obtained have already been considered in the sections on electro-physiology and electro-diagnosis. Here the electrolytic, cataphoric, vasomotor, and trophic effects will be especially considered. *Electrolysis.*—If the reader will refer to the section on Electrolysis in the first part of this work, he will there find clearly stated certain well-established laws governing the passage of the current through an electrolyte, or electrolytic conduction. These laws have been established by observation of the action of the current on inorganic compounds of simple, and hence more or less stable, composition. When we endeavor to apply these laws to the phenomena of electrolysis of organic compounds, we meet with many difficulties and apparent contradictions. There is reason to believe, however, that the laws remain the same, whether the electrolysis takes place in inorganic or organic compounds, and that the difficulty is entirely due to our deficient knowledge of what takes place when an electrolytic current is passed through organic tissue.

If we assume that organic tissues, such, for example, of which the human body is composed, are electrolytes, and that the passage of a current through such tissues always causes electrolytic decomposition, much of the difficulty vanishes. The complexity of the results of electrolysis in organic tissues as compared with inorganic electrolytes may be explained, in part at least, by the greater chemical complexity of the former. Furthermore, organic tissue—a gland, muscle, or morbid growth—must be considered as a multitude of electrolytes of different composition placed side by side; and on passing a current through such a collection of differing electrolytes we may expect not merely the results of decomposition at the electrodes, but, assuming each individual tissue (muscle-fibre, connective tissue, nerve, blood-vessel, lymph-space, etc.) to have different composition and resistances, we should have a multitude of electrodes between the two terminals of the battery, and might reasonably expect a separation of ions at each point where the current passes from one sort of tissue to another. With this conception we can understand without much difficulty what has been termed "interpolar action," but which has not heretofore been clearly explained on any physical law.

The methods of applying the galvanic current for electrolytic purposes vary with the special cases for which it is employed. Wherever applicable, one or both electrodes should be directly introduced into the tissue which it is desired to decompose. In other cases, the transmission of a current seems to be efficient, no matter whether the electrodes are directly hi contact with the tissues or not.

Electrolysis is employed for the purpose of causing absorption of serous effusions, solid inflammatory infiltrations, and new growths, for the destruction of smaller new formations (warts, noevi, tumors) or normal growths in abnormal situations (hirsuties, trichiasis). It is also taken advantage of for the destruction of the foetus in extra-uterine pregnancy. In aneurism it has taken a leading position as a safe and efficient mode of treatment, and angioma, cystic goitre, and bony ankylosis have yielded to its persistent and systematic employment.

Cataphoresis.—Various experimenters have shown that a galvanic current passing through a vessel containing fluid separated by a porous division causes a transfer of fluid through the porous partition, so that the fluid stands higher on one side of the partition than on the other. This phenomenon is called electrical osmosis. The direction of osmotic action is with the current, *i.e.,* from the anode to the cathode. Experiments upon animal tissues have shown that medicinal substances, for example, iodine, quinine, strychnine, cocaine, bichloride of mercury, etc., could be made to traverse organic tissues—the epidermis among others—in the same way. This property of the galvanic current has been taken advantage of to a limited extent to favor the entrance of medicaments through the skin. It is said that local anaesthesia has been thus produced with cocaine and chloroform, and that mercuric bichloride has in this way been "driven into" the skin and acted more efficiently as a parasiticide than when merely applied to the surface.

But it is probable that this cataphoric or osmotic action also plays a part in the action of the galvanic current in cases of serous effusion, and the absorption of infiltrations generally. While to the writer it appears probable that most of the results obtained from the galvanic current in such cases are due to the electrolytic action already referred to, it is also rational to suppose that the osmotic or propulsive action of the current assists in the removal of the morbid products.

Vasomotor Effects.—It has been already mentioned that the galvanic current produces variations in the calibre of the blood-vessels at the points of application of the electrodes. Similar modifications of the vascular calibre are produced by a stimulation of certain nerve-centres. These effects upon the vascular system are sometimes made use of for the production of therapeutic results.

Trophic Effects.—Although our knowledge of a trophic system of nerves is still very indefinite, we may assume the existence of such nerves to aid us in explaining the phenomena of nutrition. Whether galvanism has any effects upon the trophic nerves is immaterial in face of the fact that it undoubtedly has a decided influence upon nutrition. Atropines of organs or tissues are often favorably modified by the galvanic current. *Catalytic Effects.*—The effects comprised under the cataphoric, vasomotor, and trophic effects have been ascribed by R. Itemak and others to *catalytic* action. This term, which did duty for so long in chemistry until the advance of the science rendered it superfluous, has been adopted by a number of electro-therapeutists to cover our lack of definite knowledge upon the subject, Its use is only justifiable on the ground that we have no well-defined notions of what takes place when the galvanic current produces the effects spoken of. We may excuse ourselves for using the term by quoting the dictum of Mephistopheles in "Faust":—

"Wo Begriffe fehlen,
Da stellt ein Wort zur rechten Zeit sich ein;"

but its use is hardly creditable to our scientific honesty. It were better to drop it out of our technical terminology.

Special Methods of Localized Galvanization.—It has been experimentally shown by von Ziemssen and others (pp. 156, 157) that the galvanic current can be made to traverse the brain through the skull and produce decided effects. Clinical observations also seem to show that therapeutic results of value can be obtained by the transmission of electricity through this organ, not only in local cerebral complaints, but in general neuroses. The methods adopted by various electro-therapeutists for influencing the brain are the following:— (a) *Longitudinal Brain Galvanization.*—The electrodes (large, at least two inches square) are applied to the forehead and occiput, and a mild current transmitted. The electrodes should be firmly applied first and then the current gradually turned on. The current may be either stabile or labile. The points for the application of the electrodes are the median line and the frontal protuberances in front, and the occipito-vertebral junction and post-auricular space of the occiput behind. *(b) Transverse Brain Galvanization.*—Bearing in mind the physiological effects of transverse brain galvanization, *i.e.,* nausea, vertigo, etc., extreme caution is requisite in transmitting the current through the brain from side to side. Very weak currents must be employed, and by the use of a good rheostat the current will be very gradually turned on and increased to the degree necessary. The circuit should not be abruptly broken, but by increasing the resistance gradually by means of the rheostat the current should be slowly diminished to zero. It is essential for the employment of brain galvanization that a trustworthy mUliamperemeter should be in the circuit, which should be constantly watched to note the strength of the current and its increase or diminution. With the use of the electrode above mentioned, one milliampere of current is usually sufficient. The points for the application of the electrodes in transverse brain galvanization are the two sides of the frontal bone, the parietal protuberances on either side, the temporal bones, and the mastoid processes. A *stabile* current is one in which the electrodes are held firmly in the positions to which thov are applied. In the *labile* application one or both of the electrodes are moved about without raising them from the surface. *Interrupted* application consists in now and then raising one or both electrodes and reapplying thcin. This method is rarely used iu brain galvanization. (c) *Diagonal Brain Galvanization.*—In this method the same cautions should be observed as in transverse galvanization of the brain. The electrodes are applied to the frontal, frontotemporal, or fronto-parietal region on one side, and the occipital region on the other.

Sittings should never last longer than three to five minutes.

Galvanization of the brain is applicable in various neurotic and psychical disorders, *e.g.,* headache, insomnia, mental depression, aphasia, etc. These symptoms are often improved, aud in some cases the structural lesions, effusions, inflammatory infiltrations, etc., are benefited.

Spina/ Galvanization.—Galvanization of the spine may be longitudinal or transverse. In the first the electrodes are placed over the spinous processes in the cervical and the sacral regions, or short sections of the spine may be taken at a time. In transverse galvanization one pole is placed over the spine and the other applied to the median line in front. The position of the poles may be varied so that both poles may be brought successively over the scat of the lesion. Careful observation will teach the practitioner the polar effect most desirable in the case under treatment..

The current may also be transmitted from the spine to the peripheral nerves or plexuses, one electrode being placed over the spine, and the other over the respective nerve-trunk or plexus. Here, also, the current may be tried in different directions to ascertain which gives the more beneficial effect. Moderate currents, gradually increased and decreased, are indicated.

The therapeutic indications of spinal galvanization are diseases of the spinal cord, and certain functional diseases of the brain, abdominal viscera, and the generative apparatus in both sexes.

Subaural Galvanization.—This procedure, known generally as galvanization of the sympathetic, is best carried out as follows: An electrode two inches square is applied to the neck at the maxillary angle, and pressed backward toward the spine. The other electrode is applied over the transverse processes of the firth to the seventh cervical vertebra? on the opposite side of the body. A current of three to five milliamperes is used.

Although the physiological effects of such a current are indefinite, the clinical results in many cases cannot be denied.

Snbanral galvanization is used with advantage in various neuroses about the head, as migraine, insomnia, tinnitus annum, vasomotor disturbances of the brain, and various functional disorders of the digestive; and genito-urinary organs.

The methods of employing galvanization of the eye and ear have alrefldy been described on page 15o.

It may be mentioned that snbanral galvanization has been used with success in the treatment of corneal ulcer. The use of an electrode applied directly to the ulcerated surface has also been found successful. Naturally, here very mild currents are employed. In galvanization of the ear, the ear electrode before described should be used, or the current should be transmitted through a large (two-inch) electrode, applied over the mastoid process. Tinnitus aurium and nervous deafness are proper conditions for the employment of aural galvanization.

Constant Infinitesimal Currents..—The effects of apparatus kept constantly applied to the surface, such as the multifarious varieties of electric and galvanic belts, pads, brushes, combs, etc., have been studied by a number of scientific observers, but nothing very definite has been ascertained. The current furnished by these devices is so small and inconstant that they cannot be relied upon for any therapeutic effects. Notwithstanding this, however, the constant galvanic current, though minute, furnished by these arrangements may at times produce decided modifications of nutrition by electrolysis. Cases have been observed where small sloughs have formed under the battery terminals when the belts have been long worn. other there would be but slight sensory reaction to the current. The therapeutic effects would, doubtless, likewise be different. A little practical experience will show the careful observer that the electric current and its effects are not merely dependent upon the number, kind, and size of the elements employed, or upon the sort of conductors and size of the electrodes, but also upon the degree of resistance of the tissues operated upon. *Galvanic Dosage.*—Some; remarks have already been made upon this topic when discussing the measurement of currents, but the subject is of such supreme importance to the electrotherapeutist that no apology is deemed necessary for reverting to it. The older records of current strength used in diseases are not available for comparison with results obtained at the present day, except when batteries of great constancy and known electro-motive force and current were employed. We are just beginning the scientific cultivation of electro-therapeutics. The proper dosage of the current is, therefore, a subject which demands from the physician the closest attention.

As a general rule it may be accepted for our guidance at present, as deduced from clinical experience, that mild currents, other things being equal, are most desirable. Further researches in electro-therapeutics may, however, cause us to revise, if not reverse, this rule for many diseases, as the results obtained by Apostoli and his followers have already compelled us to do for one class of cases. Hence, the laws of the current, especially Ohm's law, not merely in its mathematical form, but in its daily intelligent application, must be studied by every physician who desires to succeed in the electro-therapeutic art. It must be understood, for example, that a current of 10 milliamperes is an entirely different thing in degree when the electrodes are 32 centimetres and when they are 302 centimetres in area. In the one case the sensation would be decidedly painful, while in the

Midler and Stiutzing have endeavored to indicate more particularly the proper strength of current to employ in certain diseases with definite-sized electrodes. Taking an electrode of, say, eighteen square centimetres, Midler uses a current of one milliampere as the normal standard in most cases. This is written in the form of a fraction, using the size of the electrode as a denominator and the number of milliamperes as a numerator, thus, T. Sbould he desire to use a larger electrode, say, of 362 cm., the strength of current employed is 2 ma., and the symbol is then written . £% In other cases he uses stronger currents, for example, *(i.e.,* 1 ma. and 8" cm. electrode), or, when operating about the cranium, even smaller currents, as or *fa.*

Stiutzing has shown, however, that the physiological effect of is not equivalent to *fa*; in other words, that an equal increase of current, with the size of electrode used, will lead to erroneous conclusions. He has found, for example, that-g-acts upon a motor nerve not with the strength of f, but of *fa.* Hence the symbol and fraction of Midler must not be reduced to its lowest terms, but recorded in its original form.

Stintzing states, likewise, that the currents employed by Midler are too weak for many cases. Thus he uses in spinal diseases -*§,* in brain diseases -£. :, and in subaural galvanization currents as strong as *fa.*

The general tendency of electro-therapeutists is, however, in the direction marked out by Midler, *i.e.,* weak currents and short sittings.

Duration of Sittings.—The duration of sittings is a matter that requires further study in connection with the accurate measurement of the current. In nervous disorders sittings of four or five minutes are the most usual. Midler limits the sittings generally to one-half to one minute, rarely exceeding three minutes. In obstinate neuralgias sittings of from fifteen to thirty minutes are often extremely beneficial, when shorter sittings would be ineffectual. The duration may be regulated in a measure by the strength of the current. In using a strong current, a short sitting, while with a mild current a longer sitting may be allowed. It must be distinctly understood, however, that strength of current and length of the *seance* are by no means convertible terms.

These limitations of action of electricity, both as relating to strength of current and length of sitting, are more particularly applicable when this agent is employed for brain and nervous diseases. When it comes to the use of electricity in other portions of the body, especially where definite results are looked for, as in electrolysis of uterine fibroids or other morbid growths, much stronger currents are required to produce results within a reasonable time.

Faradic Electricity.—The construction of the faradic machine (induction coil) is given in detail in the first part of this work, and special apparatuses for physicians' use are described and illustrated in Chapter III, Part II. The faradic current has a strongly-marked effect upon muscular contractility, sensation, vaso-motor conditions, and, either directly or indirectly, upon nutrition. It sometimes causes or promotes absorption of effused products, but its effects in these instances seem to depend upon a molecular disarrangement of the parts acted upon, and probably upon stimulation of the blood and lymph-vascular system, rather than upon any electrolytic effects, although some recent authors are fain to attribute a mild electrolytic effect to the faradic as well as to the galvanic current. *General Faradization.*—The method of general faradization is practically the same as that for general galvanization. One pole of the battery is connected with a plate placed under the feet or buttocks, and the other pole, armed with a large sponge electrode (or the hand of the operator may be used, as in general galvanization), is applied to the head, neck, spine, upper extremity, trunk, etc. The strength of the current can be regulated by moving the outer coil over the inner one, aided by a water rheostat in the circuit. As already shown (page 190), the current strength of a faradic machine cannot be exactly measured. The sensations or motor effects of the current must be the guide, and the coil distance will give sufficient data for record. It must not be forgotten that when the primary current is used the least current is obtained with the coils completely covering each other, and that the least current of the secondary coil is obtained when the outer coil is drawn out to its fullest extent, completely uncovering the inner coil. *Local Faradization.*—The faradic current is employed for the purpose of stimulating the skin and deeper structures. For cutaneous stimulation the brush-electrode (Fig. 199, page 238) is useful. To stimulate muscular contraction or modify nutrition in visceral organs, large metal electrodes, covered with absorbent cotton or sponge, are employed. Muscles can be stimulated through the nerves or directly through the muscular substance, if this has not undergone degeneration. (See page 203.) Muscular contraction can also be induced reflexly by cutaneous irritation of sensory nerves. This is also often effectual in disorders of the deeper-seated organs. In these cases faradism acts as a revulsive agent, producing hyperaemia of the skin and generally increased force of circulation, and thus relieving congestion of internal organs. In certain chronic hyperaemic conditions of the brain and spinal cord this method of counter-irritation with the faradic brush has given excellent results. Some electrotherapeutists limit the area of skin thus stimulated to a space of a few centimetres square, while others pass the brush over a larger surface. As a rule, the faradic brush increases cutaneous sensibility, while the use of large moist electrodes diminishes sensibility and relieves pain. In the treatment of anaesthetic conditions, therefore, the brash-electrode should be employed, and for the relief of hypenesthesia and neuralgia the sponge or cotton-covered electrode should come into play.

A method frequently giving good results in painful affections is that of " swelling faradic currents," introduced by Frommhold. The electrodes, well moistened, are applied stabile, and then the current is gradually increased, kept at its maximum for a few minutes, and then gradually decreased to zero again. This may be conveniently indicated by the symbol, Far. .

Galvano-faradization.—Beard & Rockwell, De Watteville, Stein, and others have employed the two currents in combination and have claimed special success with this method. The observations on record are not yet sufficient in number to enable us to draw definite conclusions, but the results obtained are promising. By means of a switch both currents are combined in the conducting cords, or, in some instances, in special electrodes devised for the purpose.

The combined currents are especially indicated in chronic, rheumatic swelling of the joints, with pain, atrophic paralysis, etc.

Electro-massage, by means of a roller-electrode (Fig. 206, page 239), has been used with success where a combination of electricity with the mechanical effects of massage is desirable. Chronic rheumatic joint affections and chronic inflammatory infiltrations would seem to be the best indications for this method. Either or both currents may be employed. *Frequency of Sittings.*—This depends upon the individual case and the nature of the disease. In the majority of cases, daily or semi-weekly sittings are most customary. In painful diseases—neuralgia, acute articular rheumatism, myalgia, etc.— it may be advisable to repeat the sittings several times a day. In cases of electrolysis of uterine fibroids or urethral strictures sittings once a week will usually give satisfactory results.

G A LV A NO-CAUTERY.

The galvano-cautery has decided advantages over the knife and cutting or crushing instruments, as well as over other forms of cautery in practical surgical work. In the first place, by its use haemorrhage is avoided in parts where vessels may not easily be controlled by ligature or pressure. It has the advantage over the ecraseur and snare in not tearing or pulling the tissues separated. It leaves a clean, aseptic surface which usually heals readily under the thin, dry plate of charred tissue left by the hot wire or knife. Its action can be limited as strictly as the knife or scissors, and the wire loop or burner can be applied cold to the part to be operated upon and heated when *in situ,* thus giving it a great advantage over the thermo-cautery in operations about the nose, throat, vagina, or rectum. It has the further advantage over the thermo-cautery that it radiates less heat (on account of the thinness of the heated metal). In operations about the eyes and in the nasal, oral, and vaginal cavities this is a very important point. It is the only cautery that can be used in the larynx, naso-pharynx, and urethra.

The objections to the galvano-cautery have been already pointed out (pp. 240, 241); but recent improvements in storage batteries and dynamo machines have removed many of the difficulties which surgeons had formerly to contend against when using the galvano-cautery.

Galvano-causty is applicable for the cauterization of the surface and borders of indolent or infective ulcers (tubercular, diphtheritic); the destruction of superficial new formations, as epithelioma, lupus, syphilis, naevi, etc.; the removal of small growths, as fibromata; the destruction of angioma ta; the amputation of diseased or hypertrophied organs, as the cervix uteri, clitoris, labia (elephantiasis), penis, tongue, etc.; opening abscesses, boils, or carbuncles; stimulating healthy granulations in fistulous tracts, or dividing the bridge of tissue between a fistula and the surface; removing intra-laryngeal, intra-pharyngeal,intra-nasal, and intra-utcrine growths; cauterizing exposed and painful nerves, as in carious teeth; in short, wherever the hot iron can be used to advantage over the knife, the galvanocautery should be employed.

STATIC ELECTRICITY.

The description of the static machine has been given in earlier chapters. The methods of using this form of electricity require, however, some further amplification.

Franklinization, under which term we understand the therapeutic application of static electricity, is employed by the following methods:—

Static insulation, or static charge; the indirect and direct spark; static shock, static breeze, and static induced current.

Fig. 216.—Static Insulation. *Static Insulation.*—The patient is placed upon the insulated platform, and his body, or the stool upon which he sits, connected with the machine by a chain. The chain must not touch the floor. The other pole of the machine is then grounded by attaching the chain to the gas or water fixture, or simply allowing the free end to rest upon the uncarpeted floor. The poles of the machine are now separated and the machine put in rapid motion. The patient becomes "charged" with static electricity, which escapes as he leaves the insulated platform and approaches his finger-tips to other persons or some article of furniture, or the door. Fig. 216 shows the method of performing this insulation.

Indirect and Direct Spark.—If the patient remains seated upon the platform charged as before, and a metal-hall electrode attached to a chain is connected with the gas or water fixture, sparks will be drawn from that part of the body to which the ball is approached. This is termed the "indirect spark." The "direct spark" is produced by connecting the electrode directly to the grounding-chain, so as to place the patient in a short circuit, as shown in Fig. 217. *Static Shock.*—If two Leyden jars, joined by a brass rod, be suspended from the conductors and connected, one with the platform and one with the ball-electrode, shocks are given at the approach of the electrode to the patient's body (Fig. 218).

Fig. 219.—The Electrical "head Bath." A Variety Of Administration Of The Static Breeze.

These spark applications are more or less painful, and should be used with great care. They are a powerful means of excitation of the skin as well as of the deeper organs.

Static Breeze.—If, instead of a ball-electrode, a pointed electrode of metal or wood is used, a sensation resembling a current of wind is caused. This is known as the electrical wind, spray, or breeze. When it is desired to apply this breeze to the head, a cap-shaped electrode, called an umbrella-electrode, is suspended at some distance above the patient's head (Fig. 219). *Static Induced Current.*—To produce the static induced current, a pair of sponge electrodes are connected with a couple of Leyden jars, suspended from the poles of the machine. In using this the poles should be closely approximated before applying the electrodes to the body. (See Fig. 220.) By this means a current of electricity can be sent through a nerve with a static machine, the static discharge being converted into a dynamic discharge or current of high electro-motive force.

An electrode suitable for the application of this static induced current is that devised by Dr. W. J. Morton, of New York, and termed the "pistol-electrode." It is shown in Fig. 221.

A great advantage of the static over other forms of electricity is that it can be applied through the clothing. As shown in the illustrations, sparks and sprays can be drawn from the patient through the clothing without producing any injury of the latter.

The effects of franklinization vary with the method of application and the portion of the surface to which it is applied. The gradation of effect is somewhat as follows: Static insulation is mildest in its effects, the electric breeze more decided, and the electric spark or static shock the most severe. Physiological effects of static electricity are, increase of temperature, heightened blood-pressure, more rapid circulation, increase of perspiratory and other secretions, restoration of depressed or suppressed functions (appetite, menstruation). The points of discharge of sparks (on the skin) become pale and bloodless, soon followed, however, by hyperemia. Wheals are not infrequently the result of drawing sparks from the body. Certain specific effects are produced upon the nerves of special sense; flashes when sparks are drawn from the ophthalmic region, and a vibration or hammering in the ears when applied near the ear.

Some of the best therapeutic effects of franklinization are produced in the general neuroses—hysteria, neurasthenia, insomnia, chorea, headache, etc. In all forms of neuralgia, rheumatism, spasmodic affections, and hyperesthesias the electric breeze is indicated. In anaesthesias, paralyses, morbid growths, and other conditions requiring a vigorous agitation, the direct or indirect spark and static induction are strongly indicated.

Magneto-therapy.—The medical world had almost or quite forgotten the excitement caused by the performances of Mesmer and his followers and imitators, when it was somewhat startled ten or twelve years ago by the rapidly-following announcements in scientific medical journals of Burcq, Charcot, Westphal, Onimus, Vigouroux, Rosenthal, and others, that the external application of various metals or of permanent magnets was capable of producing decided therapeutic effects. It is true that these effects were produced principally in hysterical or otherwise neurotic subjects, but the fact of their occurrence has an undoubted interest and possibly a practical value to the electro-therapeutist. It was found, for example, that laying plates of gold or other metal (coins, for example) upon the insensitive skin, in cases of hysterical hemianaesthesia, was soon followed (in ten to twenty minutes) by a return of sensation on the anaesthetic side. The first sensations were those of formication, tingling, and a sensation of warmth, gradually followed by a return of the normal sensibility. Coincident with this return of the sensibility on the affected side there was a transference of the anaesthesia to the primarily healthy side. After a time the anaesthesia returned to the primarily affected side, but could again be transferred on re-application of the metal plates.

These phenomena were subjected to a searching investigation by a commission of the French Societi de Biologie, consisting of Charcot, Luys, and Dumontpallier, and confirmed on numerous individuals. Various theories were propounded to account for the effects produced, but none of them explain the phenomena satisfactorily. It was found that magnets, when approached to the skin, produced similar effects, and that hyperaesthesia and pain could likewise be transferred from one side of the body to the other.

In pursuing these investigations certain clinical results of importance were obtained. Migraine and other forms of neuralgia, hysterical contractures, "spinal irritation," insomnia, chorea major, etc., have been treated with success by the application of the poles of a magnet wrapped in a cloth to the affected side. When the pain moves to the opposite side the magnet is also moved to that side, alternately following the pain until the latter gradually disappears. The manner in which the magnet can produce these effects is at present totally inexplicable, but, as the clinical results are vouched for by such excellent observers as Charcot, Vigouroux, Rosenthal, and Benedikt, further experimentation in this line seems indicated.

In the following pages it will frequently be noticed that diverse and apparently contradictoiy methods followed by different observers have yielded successful results. Some skeptics have cited this as an evidence that electricity is of little use in medicine because an agent that gives like results whether properly or improperly used can have little therapeutic value. Such a conclusion would be highly irrational. The fact is that our knowledge of the actions of most therapeutic agents is extremely deficient, and yet few would be willing to practice medicine without making use of the remedies whose actions we so little understand.

Every one owes it to his art to place his honest observations on record, and in course of time trustworthy conclusions may be reached respecting the therapeutic applications of electricity as in other tilings.

CHAPTER II.

Special Electro-therapeutics.

Diseases Of The Nervous System.

Diseases of the Brain.—In the electrical treatment of diseases of the brain this agent may be employed in the various forms of galvanism, faradism, galvano-faradism, franklinism, or even magneto-therapy, which may be looked upon as one method of employing electrical force.

The objects aimed at in brain electrization are modification of the vascular supply in the brain, electrolytic and trophic effects, as well as functional exaltation or depression.

In using galvanism the various methods of longitudinal, transverse, or diagonal brain galvanization may be employed. According to Lowenfeld the anode produces hyperaemia and the cathode anaemia of the side or section of the brain to which they are respectively applied. The statements of Lowenfeld are not generally accepted, however. Neftel has devised a method of labile brain galvanization which appears to have some advantages. The cathode is applied stabile to the back of the neck, and the anode passed slowly over the forehead, eyes, temple, auriculo-mastoid fossa to the mastoid region, and then back to the forehead. If required the same procedure may be repeated on the opposite side of the head. Galvanization of the medulla— one electrode to the occipito-vertebral joint and the other to the sternum or throat—and subaural galvanization may also be used. Central and general galvanization are occasionally of value. The rule should be large electrodes, weak currents (to -*fa*), and short sittings (one to two minutes).

Faradism may be employed in the form of general faradization when the current can be well controlled by the hand as one electrode. Peripheral faradization to produce reflex effects upon the intra-crauial circulation is effective. The method of Rumpf, where a large surface of the skin is stimulated, or that of Vulpian, where a very small area is subjected to the action of the faradic brush, are both valuable for their influence upon the action and nutrition of the brain.

Peripheral paralyses, spasms, contractures, and paresthesias dependent upon brain-lesions are to be subjected to local electro-therapeutical measures in accordance with general principles. The etiological factors of brain disease are to be removed, if possible, and when lesions are present that are attributable to morbid processes accessible to medical and surgical measures the latter are also to be employed. Thus, syphilitic and other morbid growths, toxic factors, etc. , require the appropriate treatment for these conditions.

Should the case, instead of improving under electricity, get worse, it is not to be concluded that the remedy is necessarily contra-indicated. Its method of application may require modification; the current may be too strong, or the sittings too long continued. If the galvanic cathode produces too much reaction the anode may be tried, or the faradic induced current may be substituted; or in place of either of these forms sUitic electricity or magneto-therapy may be employed.

The experience of various observers in the various diseases of the brain is given without comment. The writer does not venture to indicate which is the best method.

Anosmia.—Longitudinal brain galvanization, with anode over the medulla oblongata (vasomotor centre). Eulenburg advises faradization of the phrenic nerves and of the soles of the feet. *Hyperemia.*—Dry faradic brush, according to the method of Vulpian and Grasset: Strong current to a small area of the skin. The extensor surface of the forearm is recommended by these observers. Rumpf employs the brush over a larger surface, stimulating the skin of the chest, the back, and the upper extremity. Faradism to the abdomen causes rapid cerebral anaemia, sometimes so marked as to produce fainting.

Subaural galvanization, as well as longitudinal brain galvanization, cathode to vasomotor centre, may also be tried.

Cerebral Hemorrhage.—In cases of apoplexy the electrical treatment has often a good effect upon the paralyses of sensation and motion and the depressed circulation and nutrition of the paralyzed muscles. While no one will claim that brain-tissue destroyed by an effusion of blood can be restored, either by electricity or any other measure at our command, it is probable that the absorption of the effused blood can be hastened by the appropriate use of the galvanic current. There can be no doubt, also, that the reflex effects of peripheral faradic stimulation tend to promote the restoration of impaired cerebral functions. Finally, the direct trophic effects of galvanism, faradism, and static electricity upon the peripheral organs (paralyses, hyperaesthesias, anaesthesias) are generally acknowledged.

The electrical treatment of cerebral apoplexy should be begun early. If possible, the application of the galvanic current, by longitudinal, transverse, or diagonal brain galvanization, in order to secure the electrolytic action, should be begun not later than the second week after the occurrence of the lesion. Caution should, of course, be observed that the current used be sufficiently weak, and increased and decreased very gradually so as to avoid sudden shock. The rule laid down by Erb, to pass the current in the most direct line through the seat of the lesion, should be observed.

In addition to direct galvanization, subaural and spinal galvanization should be employed for their general effects. Paralyses of muscles are to be treated in accordance with the details laid down in the section on Paralysis. The faradic brush will often awaken dormant cerebral faculties, restore sensation to anaesthetic areas, and, by stimulating the circulation, improve the nutrition of paralyzed muscles. Energetic neuro-muscular faradization has similar effects.

Chronic Meningeal Inflammations, Hydrocephalus, and Sclerotic Plaques are treated by brain galvanization for the electrolytic effects', and subanral and spinal galvanization for their influence upon the general nutrition of the patient.

Cerebral Syphilis requires primarily antisyphilitic treatment, and, secondarily, the effects of electricity in promoting restoration of suspended functions (aphasia, paralysis, anaesthesia, contractures, etc.), or to remove troublesome symptoms (headache, insomnia, etc.).

DISEASES OF THE MEDULLA OBLONGATA.

Chronic Bulbar Paralysis.—Although this affection tends uniformly to a fatal termination, the testimony of the most experienced electro-therapeutists—Benedikt, Erb, Bernhardt, and Lewandowski among others—is that persistent and rational electrical treatment may temporarily arrest its progress, or, at all events, relieve troublesome symptoms. The methods are transverse galvanization of the medulla (one electrode over each mastoid process, using two to six milliamperes of current for one to two minutes), subaural and spinal galvanization, intermittent galvanization or faradization of the paralyzed muscles, forced deglutition by applying one pole to the nape of the neck and the other over the larynx and reversing the current. Faradization of phrenic nerves in cases of paralysis of the diaphragm may be used.

PSYCHOSES.

Arndt has clearly indicated the details governing the electrical treatment of psychical disturbances. Most of the more recent workers in this department have followed on the lines laid down by this distinguished alienist. The conclusions of Arndt may be summarized as follows:—

Functional psychoses are curable by electricity. Organic brain diseases accompanied by psychical disturbances may be improved in certain symptoms, but not cured.

Early resort to this treatment, especially in mild cases, gives fair promise of success.

The faradic current is useful in either primary or secondary conditions of depression. Its action is that of a general stimulant. The galvanic current is indicated in all other psychoses in which electricity is applicable. Its electrolytic, vasomotor, and trophic effects are here made available to modify the circulation and nutrition in the brain, allay excitement, and improve the general condition of the patient.

The electrical treatment of psychical disturbances naturally resolves itself into the treatment of special symptoms. The methods used with success by Arndt, Tigges, Schiile, and others are those already indicated as useful in diseases of the brain. They may conveniently be arranged in tabular form with the symptoms for which they are most appropriate:— *Symptoms. Methods of Electrization.* f Galvanization of the brain and medulla;

Insomnia, general faradization; subaural and spinal

I-galvanization; static electricity.
M ELANCHOLY, HYPOCHONDRIA, Stupor,....

Brain, subaural, and spinal galvanization; central galvanization; general faradization and localized applications of the faradic . brush (method of Vulpian); static electricity.

Katatonia, Headache, J Brain and spinal galvanization; general Precordial Pressure,.) faradization; faradization of phrenic nerve.

Hysterical And Reflex
Psychosis, Beoinning

Stages Of Progressive
Paralysis,....

Galvanization of the brain; general faradization; subaural, spinal, and central galvanization; static electricity.

Hallucinations Of Sight J Localized galvanization, with anode to And Hearing,...) affected organ.

GENERAL NEUROSES.

Neurasthenia.—Static electricity, especially the static charge, is indicated in this condition. General faradization, especially the faradic brush in cases with much depression, and central, subaural, spinal, and brain galvanization, and electric baths in conditions of excitement or irritability. In spinal neurasthenia or "spinal irritation" galvanization with the anode to the painful points, local franklinization (static breeze), and the faradic brush have been successful. Sexual neurasthenia requires, in addition to appropriate moral treatment, faradic baths; spinal, subaural, and vagus galvanization, galvano-faradization, and electro-massage. *Hypochondria.*—General faradization and faradic baths, static insulation, and faradic brush over the chest and the upper extremities are the indicated measures. Special symptoms, as constipation, insomnia, and sexual disturbances, should receive appropriate attention. *Hysteria.*—General faradization, general and central galvanization, faradic baths, and brain, subaural, and spinal galvanization are indicated. The static breeze is also employed with success. Anode application to painful points along the spine has a favorable influence upon the general condition.

It is important, as pointed out by Erb, to gain the confidence of the patient, otherwise the treatment is likely to fail. Weak currents and short sittings should be the rule.

The psychical element in all cases of hysteria renders it extremely difficult to determine how much of the effect of treatment, if any, is to be attributed to the electricity and how much to the influence exerted upon the imagination. Ultimately this makes really very little difference, as most other remedies used against this disease are open to the same criticism.

The special or local manifestations of hysteria usually yield more easily to electricity than does the general hysterical condition. In ovaralgia, Hoist has recently indicated a method which has been successful. The anode is placed over the spine and the cathode over the painful ovary. The faradic current may be used in like manner.

Other painful points occurring in hysteria (hysterogenic points of Richter) may be treated with either current. These points are found most frequently along the dorsal spine, in the left hypochondriac and infra-mammary regions, and at spots on the front of the abdomen.

Hysterical paralyses must be treated in accordance with the usual methods in these affections. (See page 293 *et seq.*) Hysterical aphonia often yields with the greatest promptness to transverse faradization of the larynx (percutaneous), or by one electrode being introduced into the pharynx and the other applied over the thyroid cartilage. Transverse brain galvanization has been found effectual in hysterical aphonia by Emminghaus.

Anaesthesia and hemianaesthesia yield to the faradic brush (by Vulpian's method), static breeze, and occasionally to magnetotherapy.

Hysterical vomiting may be treated by applying the faradic brush to the pit of the stomach. Constipation and tympanites (phantom tumor) are sometimes relieved by energetic faradization of the abdomen as well as by static electricity.

Spasms and contractures may be treated with either current, or with static electricity, but the successes are not very numerous. Hystero-epileptic attacks can sometimes be broken up by a strong galvanic or faradic current.

Epilepsy.—Erb, in whose opinion the changes upon which epilepsy depends are located in the cortical area of the brain, advocates diagonal, followed by longitudinal, brain galvanization to affect the supposed lesion directly; then subaural and spinal galvanization limited to the cervical region, and general faradization for their reflex and generally stimulant effects. He claims to have had favorable results with this course continued for a long time between the attacks, and in combination with the usual medicinal and hygienic remedies. *Exophthalmic Goitre.*—This curious disease is now generally considered as a neurosis. Of the characteristic symptoms, excessive frequency of the pulse, enlargement of the thyroid gland, and prominence of the eyeballs, the two former are distinctly influenced by electrical treatment. Chvostek, Eulenburg, and others have reported cases in which very favorable Tesults were obtained. The pulse is often greatly lessened in frequency, being reduced ten to twenty beats per minute. This effect is not permanent, but on frequent repetition of the sittings some durable effects are often obtained. Erb recommends spinal galvanization, transverse and diagonal brain galvanization to affect the medulla oblongata, subaural and vagus galvanization. To modify the exophthalmos, one pole is placed over the closed eye and the other in the auriculo-maxillary fossa, or the current is passed transversely through the orbits. General faradization and electric baths have also been used. Rockwell, in addition to methods above mentioned, advises the application of the cathode to the sternum, and anode over the solar plexus. Faradization of the sympathetic has been successfully employed by Katyschew. The enlarged thyroid is treated by transverse galvanization, or by applying one electrode, preferably the cathode, over the gland, and the other in the auriculo-maxillary angle. Transverse galvanization or faradization of the heart (from sternum to spine) is also used to reduce the rapidity of the pulse. The faradic brush over the cardiac region is also recommended. Weak currents (V-5V) ana" short sittings should be the rule. Many sittings—Erb says thirty to one hundred—are required to produce good effects.

Chorea.—Brain, subaural, spinal, and central galvanization, general faradization, and local static applications have been used. with success. Most authorities recommend weak currents, but M. Meyer and Leube use strong interrupted currents. *Athetosis.*—When idiopathic, brain, subaural, and central galvanization, and currents from spinal cord to peripheral muscles are indicated. *Vertigo.*—Galvanization and faradization of the brain, and faradic brush to trunk and upper extremities may be tried. If there is a tendency to one-sided vertigo the cathode should be applied to that side of the head toward which the patient falls. *Tremor.*—General faradization and electric baths; central galvanization; local faradization of the trembling limbs. The results are very uncertain. In paralysis agitans no permanent good results have been obtained. Electric baths have been found useful by Eulenburg. Static charge and sparks have been used by Charcot. Transverse brain galvanization has also been recommended. *Tetanus.*—The at present accepted pathology of tetanus as an infectious disease would seem to preclude the hope of obtaining any good results from the electric current, but some observations on record, indicate that spinal galvanization with galvanization of the peripheral muscles has a quieting effect upon the spasms. Mendel has reported success in two cases. *Tetany.*—In this disease there is increase of electrical irritability. The treatment indicated is galvanization of the spine and peripheral nerve-trunks. The anode to the spine has given good results during the attacks (Erb, Eisenlohr). Careful faradization of the spine with large, moist electrodes may also be useful. *Writers', Telegraphers', and Piano-players' Cramp, and Other Forms of Co-ordination Neuroses.*—Erb has laid down the rule that in these cases the entire cerebro-spinal nervous system from centre to periphery should be subjected to systematic electrization. First, there should be brain, subaural, and spinal galvanization; then galvanization of the peripheral nerves and muscles. Faradization of the affected muscles should also be resorted to. All electrical treatment should be combined with massage and rest of the overtaxed muscles.

DISEASES OF THE SPINAL CORD AND ITS MEMBRANES.

The agreement is general among neurologists that the electrical treatment of diseases of the spinal cord offers more prospect of cure, or at least of relief of symptoms, than any other method of treatment at our command. It must be admitted that success with this therapeutic measure is far from constant, but without it we are nearly powerless against most of the grave affections that attack this important organ.

The methods in most general use are longitudinal and transverse galvanization of the spine, subaural galvanization, the faradic brush, and static electricity in its various methods of application. Sittings should not last over three minutes, and in direct galvanization of the cord currents of j to should not be used unless in exceptional cases, when voltaic alternatives may also be employed. In the "system diseases" of the cord, posterior and lateral scleroses, and in multiple sclerosis, in which the cord is diseased for a considerable portion of its length, longitudinal galvanization (one electrode in the cervical region, the other over the sacrum) is rationally indicated in order that the current may traverse the entire extent of the organ affected. The two electrodes may be moved up and down alternately in order to get the benefit of the polar effects of the current.

When but a short segment of the spinal cord is involved in the disease, as in transverse myelitis, transverse galvanization would seem to be the better method. One electrode is applied over the spine and the other on the median line of the trunk in front. Here the poles may also be reversed with good effect.

In certain cases of spinal disease there are painful pressure points over the spinous processes. These are treated by applying the anode stabile over the spot, the cathode being placed at an indifferent point.

Chronic Spinal Meningitis and Pachymeningitis.—After the irritative symptoms have subsided, spinal galvanization for its vasomotor and electrolytic effects is indicated. Atrophies and paralyses of muscles demand localized electrization. *Meningeal Haemorrhage.* —Spinal galvanization, either longitudinal or transverse, to promote electrolysis and absorption of the effused blood. *Spinal Congestion and Spinal Irritation.*—These conditions must be treated cautiously with weak galvanic currents. The faradic brush (Vulpian's method, *i.e.,* stimulation of limited areas) and faradic baths are often followed by very excellent results. *Spinal Apoplexies and Injuries of the Cord.*— Localized spinal galvanization, longitudinal and transverse. *Chronic Myelitis.* —Chronic inflammation of the spinal cord presents itself in several forms, but the transverse and compression myelitis, in consequence of vertebral caries, most frequently comes under the care of the practitioner. In these cases, direct galvanization, longitudinal and transverse, of the affected portion of the cord, is the rationally indicated procedure. While the results are somewhat uncertain, many cases are decidedly improved, and some permanently cured. It is evident that the only effect of the current to be striven after in these cases is the electrolytic or absorptive, and hence the application of faradism or static electricity cannot be expected to be of much benefit. *Multiple and Lateral Scleroses.*—In these, still rather obscure affections of the spinal cord, little permanent effect can be expected from electrical treatment, but Erb, E. Remak, Midler, and others have reported successes which should stimulate others to greater exertions. Spinal and subaural galvanization are indicated, and in multiple sclerosis peripheral farado-cutaneous stimulation with the faradic brush are suggested by E. Remak and Rumpf. In lateral sclerosis (spastic spinal paralysis), faradism should be avoided. *Locomotor Ataxia (Tabes Dorsalis, Posterior Sclerosis).*—The electrical treatment of this prevalent and grave disease of the spinal cord gives excellent results when carefully and properly carried out. Benedikt, von Krafft-Ebing, R. and E. Remak, Erb, M. Meyer, Rosenthal, Rumpf, Seeligmidler, Lewandowski, and numerous others report, not only relief from troublesome symptoms, but positive and complete cures. Rumpf reports, among twenty-four cases, four completely cured, ten greatly improved, and only one unimproved. Lewandowski, one hundred and twenty cases, twelve (10 per cent.) cured, 80 per cent. improved in one or more of the impaired functions. The improvement continued for several months or years.

The methods used are: Spinal galvanization, with galvanization or faradization of the peripheral nerves. Subaural galvanization, and static electricity to the spine. Painful points are treated by placing the cathode over the painful area, and the anode over the corresponding nerve-root. Lancinating pains and the girdle symptom are treated in the same manner. Rumpf lauds highly the application of the dry faradic brush to the trunk and extremities for ten-minute sittings daily, or even-other day. The static spark is highly recommended in the lightning pains by Ranney. Swelling i'aradic currents (Far.) are also useful in the same symptoms. Symptoms referable to the eyes, ears, extremities, bladder, etc., are to be treated by localized electrization according to the methods described in their appropriate places in this work.

Poliomyelitis.—The sufferers from the various diseases due to lesions of the anterior columns of the spinal cord, such as acute infantile paralysis, atrophic spinal paralysis, and progressive muscular atrophy, are not particularly favorable subjects for electrical treatment, but cases of improvement, and even of cure, have been reported. It is desirable to continue studying the effects of this agent upon this very grave class of cases. Electromassage and galvano-faradization are to be added to the methods above recommended for other diseases of the cord.

DISTURBANCES OF SENSATION.

Neuralgia.—Erb defines neuralgia as consisting of "pains of great intensity and peculiar quality, which arise spontaneously, are restricted to one or more areas of nerve-distribution, are felt over the entire area of distribution of the affected nerve. and manifest distinct exacerbations, remissions, or even intermissions."

The causes of neuralgia should always be sought after before beginning treatment. Traumatic, neurotic, rheumatic, reflex, and toxic causes can generally be made out. Treatment is usually more effective if the etiology of the affection is clear.

The indications for the electrical treatment of neuralgia are: 1. To bring into action the electrolytic, vasomotor, and trophic effects of the current by the application of both poles over the seat of the lesion (if this is known). 2. The calmative effect: anode over painful spots, and cathode over the point of origin of the nerve or the plexus. The reverse position of the poles is probably equally or more successful. 3. To obliterate the painful sensation by a momentary greater impression (reflex action).

The anode treatment of painful spots (Valleix's points) is often followed by complete cessation of the neuralgia. Sittings may require to be prolonged for ten minutes, although three to five minutes are usually sufficient. The electrodes should be large, well-moistened, and firmly fixed to the part in order not to vary the resistance until cessation of the pain. The current should then be gradually diminished to zero, in order to avoid the shock of a closing contraction when the electrodes are removed.

At times the reverse method must be adopted, and the cathode applied to the painful points, or directly to the painful area. V. A. may be used. Faradization of the nerve with a large, moist electrode, or the faradic brush according to Rumpf 's method are useful. Local static electricity has favorable results to its.credit, while constant. weak currents, galvano-puncture with the cathode, and the cathodic application to the skin with a metallic plate may occasionally lead to success.

In general neuroses accompanied by neuralgia, general and central galvanization and faradization, electrical baths, brain and subaural galvanization are all useful.

The cataphoric employment of the current with cocaine, aconite,and chloroform has been used to relieve pain in neuralgia.

Special neuralgias require more specific directions for treatment.

Trifacial Neuralgia (Tic Dou/ourjux).— The anode application to the painful points should be first tried. If this fails, the anode may be applied to the back of the neck, and the cathode over the painful area, or the point of emergence of the nerve or branch from the bony canals. Swelling faradic currents may be tried, or the faradic pencil to the neck. The static breeze has been found effectual in cases where other forms of electrical application had failed. Severe cases of *tic* may be temporarily improved by the electrical treatment, but permanent cures are rarely obtained. The reasons for this lack of success is that the lesion of the nerve is often located deeply in the bony canals, where it is inaccessible to the electric current. In some obstinate cases, where temporary relief follows the application, several sittings a day may prove beneficial.

Cervico-occipital Neuralgia.—The painful spots in this form of neuralgia are found "(1) midway between the mastoid process and the spine, at the point at which the great occipital nerve becomes superficial; (2) over the branches of the cervical plexus between the sterno-mastoid and trapezius; and (3) just above the parietal eminence, the focus common to occipital and trigeminal neuralgia."

The nerve is accessible throughout nearly its entire extent. Anode treatment of painful points may, if unsuccessful, be varied with galvanization of the nerve, or faradization, either with moist electrodes or the faradic moxa. Static breeze directed to the neck for five minutes daily may also be tried.

Migraine.—True hemicrania is not a favorable condition for electrical treatment. Few successes are obtained either with the galvanic or faradic current.

Cervico-brachial Neuralgia.—Painful spots are found in the following localities: in the axilla (axillary), at the posterior border of the deltoid (circumflex), behind the elbow (superior ulnar), in front of the wrist (inferior ulnar), by the side of the inferior cervical spines (vertebral), at the inferior angle of the shoulder-blade (scapular), on the outer side of the arm, three

Gowers, Dis. of the Nervous System. Phila., 1888.

inches above the condyle (external humeral), and in the lower and outer part of the forearm (radial).

The galvanic current (anode to painful points), including galvanization of the cervical spine, the brachial plexus, and the nerve-trunks. Faradization with moist electrodes, or the faradic brush. Very favorable results are often obtained..

Dorso-intercostal Neuralgia.—The etiology of dorso-intercostal neuralgias is of considerable prognostic importance. In the rheumatic, neurotic or traumatic forms, success is frequently and promptly obtained; but when the pain is due to vertebral caries, tumors, phthisis, or locomotor ataxia, little benefit can be hoped for from electrical treatment. The locations of the *points douloureux* are well known—by the sides of the vertebrae, in the mid-axillary line, and near the middle line in front.

The same methods of treatment as-are appropriate for other forms of neuralgia may be adopted: anode applications to painful points; faradization and galvano-faradization; static breeze. The prognosis is most favorable in rheumatic cases.

Lumbo-abdominal and Genito-crural Neuralgia. — "Foci of pain and tender points are found at the back beside the vertebrae, over the posterior branches; at the middle of the iliac crest (iliac point); at the lower part of the rectus (hypogastric point); while sometimes there is in the male a *scrotal* and in the female a *labial point."* f

The treatment must be conducted on the same principles: spinal galvanization; anode treatment of painful points with the cathode over the nerve-roots; or reversal of the poles. The static breeze has also been used with success, as has the faradic brush.

Sciatica.—True neuralgia of the sciatic nerve is rare, the frequent pain along the course of this nerve being in nearly all cases neurotic. There is generally pain throughout the entire course of the nerve.

The following painful spots are enumerated by Gowers: Gowers, *Inc. cit.* t Gowers, *loc. cit.* "lumbar, near the spine, just above the sacrum; *sacro-iliac,* at the articulation of the same name; a *gluteal,* opposite the middle of the lower border of the gluteus; a series of spots, varying in exact position along the course of the nerve in the posterior aspect of the thigh; a *peroneal,* behind the head of the fibula; a *malleolar,* behind the lower extremity of the fibula, and an *external plantar,* at the outer border of the foot."

In recent cases, especially of the neurotic and rheumatic forms, electrical treatment is nearly always followed by success. The methods are: Stabile galvanization of the nerve by sections; anode application to painful points; faradization with wet electrodes and with the dry brush; faradic moxa over the point of exit of the nerve; electropuncture; static breeze and sparks, and strong labile galvanic currents.

Articular Neuroses.—(See *Diseases of Muscles and Joints.*)

ANAESTHESIA.

The loss of function of the sensory nerves may be due to inflammation, compression, traumatism, or other interruption in the transmissibility of sensory impressions. In the majority of cases it yields very promptly to the influence of the electric current. The methods of applying electricity in anaesthesia are: Galvanism of the brain and spinal cord, localized galvanization and faradization,—the latter, especially, by means of the faradic brush, according to the methods of Vulpian and of Rumpf. The galvanic brush, faradic moxa, static insulation, breeze, and sparks, and magneto-therapy, as well as in some cases galvanofaradization, are indicated. When the galvanic current is employed the anode should be placed over the nerve-root, and the cathode to the anaesthetic area, for the indication is to produce excitation of the skin.

Trigeminal Anwsihesia.—Transverse brain galvanization; galvanization of the trunk and branches of the fifth nerve; the faradic brush to the anaesthetic surface, or to a small area of the forearm, as indicated by Vulpian. *Anasstlwsia of the Larynx and Pharynx.*—The application of the faradic current by means of an intra-pharyugcal insulated electrode is sometimes practiced, but percutaneous application seems to be equally effective. Intermittent galvanization may also be employed. *Hysterical Anaesthesia and Hemiancesthesia.*—The method of Vulpian (dry faradic brush to a small area on the extensor surface of the forearm) gives good results. Central galvanization, and brain and spinal galvanization, should also be practiced. If painful spots are found along the spine, or the ovaries are tender upon pressure, the anode application of the galvanic current should be employed. Where other means fail, the static breeze or sparks may be tried. *Hemianaesthesia,* due to central or toxic causes, very frequently yields promptly to the application of the faradic brush according to Vulpian's method. *Tabetic Ancesthesia.*—This is rarely permanently relieved. In addition to the farado-cutaneous brush (according to the methods of either Vulpian or ltumpf) spinal galvanization should be employed. *Traumatic Anaesthesia of the Extremities.*—Galvanization, interrupted and stabile, of the nerve-trunks and branches involved. Faradization with moist electrodes or the dry brush.

SPASMS AND CONTRACTURES.

Hyperkinetic conditions of nerves and muscles do not yield to electricity as do the analogous neuralgias. In some cases, however, the results of persistent electrical treatment are brilliant. In rheumatic contractures the electrolytic and trophic effects of the galvanic current should be sought. In spasms such as tic convulsif, blepharospasm, nictitation, etc., when not symptomatic of local inflammatory trouble, painful points along the course of the affected nerves should be subjected to the anode application. The current should be mild) and continued for from three to five minutes daily. When the cause of the spasms is centric, brain and subaural galvanization are indicated.

In reflex spasms, the anode treatment of the reflex centre (medulla oblongata) may be successful. Swelling faradic currents, and in some cases the faradic brush to the nape of the neek as a counter-irritant, are sometimes employed.

Spasms of the Face.—The muscles supplied by the motor nerves of the face are subject to spasmodic contractions, varying in extent and due to a variety of causes. In masticatory or vocal spasm, tic convulsif, blepharospasm, spasms of the eyemuscles, etc., when the cause is centric, brain, subaural, and spinal galvanization, followed by galvanization of the affected nerve-trunk, are indicated. *Spasms of the Muscles Supplied by the Spinal Accessory Nerve.*—Painful points when present should be treated by the stabile anode application of the galvanic current. Galvanization of the brain, medulla oblongata, and cervical spine may also be employed. Galvanization and faradization of the affected muscles give excellent results in rheumatic torticollis. Swelling faradic applications repeated several times a day are particularly successful in this common affection. The static breeze or spark (locally) is also a favorite method with some electrotherapeutists. *Spasms of the Respiratory Muscles (Singultus, Sneezing, Coughing, Nervous Cough, etc.).*—According to Erb, energetic faradization (dry brush) of the epigastrium is the best treatment. Galvanization of the phrenic nerves may also be used. In sneezing, galvanization of the nasal mucous membrane,— by filling the nostrils with water and introducing one electrode, the other being placed over the back of the neck or applied to the sternum. In spasms of the laryngeal muscles, transverse faradization and galvanization of the larynx are frequently beneficial. *Spasms of the Upper and Lower Extremities.*—These are often due to morbid conditions of the motor area of the brain, and may be relieved by appropriate metbods of brain galvanization.. When due to peripheral nerve-lesions (inflammation, scars, etc.), the electrolytic effects of the galvanic current should be brought into requisition. Joint troubles, causing spasms or contractures, require the methods of treatment appropriate in the case. Painful spots over the course of the nerves may often be relieved by stabile anode applications, or galvanization of the spine. Some electro-therapeutists claim good results from faradization of the antagonists of the contractured muscles. This method may be adopted in cases where the procedures above indicated have failed.

PARALYSIS.

Erb states the object of electrical treatment of paralysis to be "the restoration of the normal power of the will over the muscles, which means, in the majority of cases, the restoration of conduction in the motor-nerve tracts; and in a smaller proportion of cases the restoration of the irritability, contractility, and nutrition of the muscles. In all cases, the alterations in the nerves and muscles consequent upon the paralysis are also to be removed."

Paralysis may be divided into two general classes: *neuropathic,* in which the lesion is situated in the brain, spinal cord, or peripheral nerves; and, *myopathic,* when the lesion is in the muscle-substance itself.

Referring the reader to the text-books on diseases of the nervous system for a full exposition of the pathology, symptoms, and causation of the various palsies, the discussion in this place will be restricted to the electrical treatment of these affections.

The methods naturally vary somewhat with the seat and character of the lesion. In cases depending upon cerebral lesions, longitudinal, transverse, and diagonal brain galvanization, already described, will be brought into requisition. When the lesion is in the spinal cord, spinal galvanization in its various forms will be employed, and where the cause of the palsy is in the peripheral nerves these will be subjected to the influence of the galvanic current. In myopathic palsies, likewise, the stimulating influence of galvanism will be made use of. In addition to the galvanic current, faradism is also useful, especially in cases where the farado-muscular contractility is. preserved. The reflex effect of cutaneous faradization with the dry brush is likewise made available in the treatment of laralyzed muscles. Static charge and sparks are recommended by some authorities.

Electronicrapie, 2te aufl., p. 333. Leipzig, 1886.

Before beginning the electrical treatment of a case of paralysis, a positive diagnosis of the nature and seat of the lesion upon which the loss of motility depends is imperatively necessary. Here electricity comes in as an aid, for the reactions of the paralyzed muscles to the current indicate the nature or seat of the lesion. For example, in central palsies, there is at first an increase of electrical irritability which later becomes normal, but there is no reaction of degeneration. The latter is, however, an attendant upon paralyses of peripheral origin.

In Part II, Chapter II, the characteristics of the reaction of degeneration have been considered at some length. The phenomena of It. 1). are, however, so closely interwoven with the prognosis of certain paralyses that their clinical significance and relations to the gravity of the case may be stated as follows:—

"1. The faradic and galvanic irritability of the nerve and muscle (each examined singly) is preserved unchanged in spite of complete motor paralysis. This may be the rase in cerebral as well as in light peripheral palsies. If cerebral paralysis can be excluded on other grounds the diagnostic-prognostic conclusion would be as follows: Light peripheral paralysis, which will last about three or four weeks. Electrical treatment unnecessary.

"2. Complete motor paralysis; faradic and galvanic irritability of the nerve diminished to a greater or less degree; the faradic irritability of the muscle is diminished or abolished, while the galvanic irritability is increased. The galvanic contraction is slow and the anode closing contraction is equal to or exceeds the cathode closing contraction (partial R. D.). The muscle is very little or not at all atrophied. Diagnostic-prognostic conclusion: Moderate paralysis of neuritic character. In peripheral cases the prognosis is favorable. The paralysis may continue from one to five months.

"3. Absolute motor palsy; complete reaction of degeneration of the early stage, moderate atrophy of the muscle. The nervous irritability for both currents is abolished. The faradomuscular irritability is entirely abolished, while the galvanic irritability of the muscle is increased. The galvano-muscular contraction is always of a slow, tardy character, and generally (but not always) the normal formula of contraction is reversed, so that the An. Cl. C. is equal to or greater than the Ca. Cl. C. Diagnostic-prognostic conclusion: Grave paralysis lasting in the most favorable case five to ten months. Curability of the paralysis may be expected onlyr when the paralyzed muscles show evidences of return of trophic or motor innervation.

"4. Absolute motor palsy; complete reaction of degeneration of late stage, extreme atrophy of the muscle. Galvanic and faradic irritability of the nerve abolished. Faradic irritability of the muscle absent, but galvanic contractility weak, and only produced by strong currents, and, finally, only on application of voltaic alternatives. The muscle is reduced to a cord in size, and hard. Diagnostic-prognostic conclusion; Extreme degree of paralysis, lasting at least ten to twelve months. The probability of cure diminishes with the length of time during which these phenomena continue. Signs of restoration of function or nutrition of the nerve increase the probability of a return of the normal function of the paralyzed part."

Duchenne has called attention to a hyperasthetic condition of the paralyzed muscles which comes on in the course of the faradic treatment. This muscular hyperesthesia is a valuable Von Zieinsscn, Die Elektrkitiit in der Mcilicin, 5te aufl. Berlin, 1887.

prognostic indication of the impending return of trophic and motor innervation. Von Ziemssen agrees with the French author in considering this symptom of value, but states that its absence is not in all cases an unfavorable prognostic.

SPECIAL PARALYSES.

Facial Palsy (Bell's Palsy).—This most

common of all forms of peripheral palsies (Fig. 222) isually yields very promptly to electrical treatment. In the milder cases, where there is no R. D., or where this is only partial, the prognosis is favorable,

Fig. 222.—Bell's Paralysis. (After Ranney.) the normal contractility of the muscles being usually restored within two months. The severer forms, with complete R. D., sometimes yield after months of persistent electrical treatment, but the prognosis in such cases is not hopeful.

The diagnosis between central and peripheral paralysis, which is readily made by the" electrical reaction, should always be established before beginning treatment, as it will save much disappointment to both physician and patient.

The results aimed at in electrical treatment are two: (1) to remove the inflammatory products in and around the track of the nerve through the electrolytic effects of the current, and ('2) to limit or arrest atrophy, contracture, or spasm of the muscles by stimulating the normal nutritive process.

The methods of treatment to be followed in Bell's paralysis are as follow: Transverse occipital brain galvanization and subaural galvanization. This is followed by galvanization of the nervetrunk and its branches; faradization of the nerve, one pole being placed over the stylo-mastoid foramen and the other successively over the motor points of the paralyzed muscles. Static electricity (breeze and sparks) may be applied along the course of the nerve. Galvanofaradization may also be used, especially in obstinate cases. The faradic brush over the area of distribution of the sensory branches of the fifth nerve may sometimes bring about contraction of the paralyzed muscles by reflex action.

The electrical treatment should be begun as early as possible after the lesion, in order to prevent contracture.

Facial paralysis of central origin offers a much more serious prognosis. Recoveries are comparatively rare, although decided improvement sometimes follows electrical treatment. Tbe centric methods of electrization, brain and subaural galvanization, must not be omitted in this variety of palsy. The paralyses of the muscles of mastication generally belong to the centric palsies, and must be treated upon the principles already laid down for affections of central origin.

In paralysis of the eye-muscles the lesion is usually peripheral. Galvanic and faradic stimulation are indicated. When the former is employed, the anode is placed over the back of the neck, and the cathode to the closed lids. Or a very fine electrode may be used to stimulate the muscles through the motor points found on the bulbar side of the lids. In mydriasis either the galvanic or faradic currents may be used. In using the former, mild currents and small electrodes are employed, the anode being placed over the middle of the closed eye, and the cathode swept around the orbital border. The faradic current may be applied directly to the conjunctiva after benumbing the sensation with cocaine. *Paralysis of the Spinal Accessory.—* Tins affects principally the sterno-cleido-mastoid and trapezius muscles. The methods of treatment indicated are spinal galvanization and galvanic or faradic stimulation of the paralyzed muscles, and the faradic brush to the skin over the muscles. The lesion in the nerve is usually peripheral, and the prognosis is favorable. If the paralysis is of central origin, brain galvanization should be added to the other procedures mentioned. *Hypoglossal Paralysis.—* Transverse brain galvanization, and intermittent galvanic stimulation of the muscles of the tongue. The cathode is applied to the motor point for the hypoglossal nerve, and the anode to the back of the neck. This form of paralysis is frequently an accompanying symptom of brain or medullar lesions. *Paralysis of the Muscles of Deglutition.—* This is a frequent sequel of diphtheria, and should be treated principally with galvanization and faradization of the muscles of deglutition. Anode to back of the neck, cathode to cheeks and lips, or faradization of the velum, will often cause attempts at swallowing. *Laryngeal Paralysis.—*In addition to galvanization of the brain and cervical spine, percutaneous faradization and galvanization are indicated. Intra-laryngeal electrization is difficult to perform. When it is desired to stimulate the laryngeal muscles directly, an insulated urethral sound may be used. Von Ziemssen has devised a double electrode for intra-laryngeal use, but this method is rarely employed, equally good or better effects being secured from the percutaneous applications of the current. Erb advises the anode to be placed on the back of the neck well up under the occiput, and the cathode to be passed up and down along the front of the larynx and trachea in order to bring all the laryngeal muscles and nerves under the influence of the current. Faradism may be employed in the same way. *Paralysis of the Upper Extremity.—*In the palsies of the various muscles of the upper extremity the galvanic current is employed to influence the appropriate nerves from the spine to the plexus, and then along the course of the various nervetrunks. In cases of traumatic paralysis the current should be passed directly through the seat of the injury in order to obtain the electrolytic and trophic effects. Faradism is used either with large, moist electrodes, to stimulate the muscles directly, or by the dry faradic brush to obtain reflex contractions. *Paralysis of the Muscles of the Trunk.—*To stimulate the serratus muscle the anode is applied to the cervical spine, and the cathode to the long thoracic nerve in the supra-clavicular fossa, in the axilla, and along the course of the nerve. The faradic current may be employed in the same way. The muscles of the abdomen and loins are directly stimulated by both galvanic and faradic currents. Large electrodes and strong currents should be used to obtain decided contractions. *Paralysis of the Lower Extremity.—*In the paralyses of the thigh-or leg-muscles the galvanic current is employed from the spine, especially the lower portion, to the plexuses, nervetrunks, and muscles. Faradization of the muscles is also useful. In all the varieties of motor paralysis, static electricity in the form of the static breeze or sparks may also be employed. *Diphtheritic Paralysis.*—The muscles of the trunk and extremities and the heart are sometimes paralyzed or in a paretic condition as a result of diphtheria. Severe attacks of other infectious diseases sometimes leave similar effects. In all these cases brain and spinal galvanization, with direct application of the current to the affected muscles, should be tried. The heart may be galvanized by direct transmission of the current from the back to the sternum. Large electrodes and mild currents should be used, and the current should be frequently reversed (seventy to eighty times per minute). Static electricity has also been used with good effect. *Syphilitic Paralysis.*—Paralysis from syphilitic infiltrations should be treated with local and general galvanization and faradization, in conjunction with appropriate specific treatment. *Toxic Paralyses,* from lead, mercury, or other poisons, require not only peripheral application of the galvanic and faradic currents, but also spinal galvanization, especially in the cervical portion of the cord, and from the nape of the neck to the sternum. Static electricity is also useful. *Muscular Paralyses and Atrophies* from disuse, or idiopathic disease of the muscles should be subjected to local faradization and galvanization.

DISEASES OF THE PERIPHERAL NERVES.

Neuritis and Perineuritis.—Galvanism through the affected portion of the nerve, or the faradic brush, or moxa, and faradomassage are indicated. In recent cases the anode is placed over the seat of the lesion and the cathode in a convenient position near by, so that the current will pass with more or less directness through the lesion.

DISEASES OF THE SYMPATHETIC SYSTEM.

The methods of electrization used in abnormal conditions supposed to be due to disease of the sympathetic nervous system are, principally, subaural galvanization ("galvanization of the sympathetic") and galvanization of the cervical portion of the spinal cord. Strong currents and voltaic alternatives are sometimes indicated. In cutaneous angioneuroses (angiospasm, angioparcsis) the employment of general faradization, subaural galvanization, and local faradization and galvanization are appropriate methods of treatment. When the vessels are contracted direct faradic application by brush or moist electrode with strong currents produces dilatation. Weak currents of short duration with the moist electrodes to the part, or the dry faradic brush on the opposite side of the body, produce contraction of the vessels.

Angina Pectoris.—In the attack the application of strong faradic currents through the faradic brush to the precordial region has produced prompt relief. Subaural and spinal galvanization are also recommended in the intervals between the attack. Transverse galvanization of the heart (von Ziemssen's method) may be tried. *Palpitation of the Heart.*—In this affection the same methods as are employed in angina pectoris are indicated. In weak, dilated heart von Ziemssen has seen good effects from strong galvanic currents passed through the heart from the front to the back of the chest, with frequent reversal of the current (V. A.). *Nervous Asthma.*—Subaural and spinal galvanization, with transverse laryngeal galvanization and faradization, are sometimes useful. Subaural galvano-faradization may also be employed. Faradization of the pneumogastric is recommended by De Watteville and others.

DISEASES OF THE MUSCLES AND JOINTS.

In diseases of the organs of locomotion electricity is often of very great value. The methods of application consist principally of local galvanization and faradization, although in some affections the various methods of central electrization are also useful.

Pseudo-hypertrophy of Muscles and Thomsen's Disease (Myotonia Congenita).—Neither of these affections give much promise of success to the electrical treatment, but Erb advises general faradization, electric baths, and galvanization of the muscles, with central galvanization. *Myalgia (Muscular Rheumatism).*—Few diseases yield more promptly and completely to electricity than the various forms of acute muscular rheumatism. Lumbago, rheumatic torticollis, pleurodynia, etc., often disappear like magic (" wie weggeblasen "), as Erb says, after the application of the dry faradic brush over the painful muscle for a few minutes. Strong currents, sufficient to redden the skin, are required. If necessary the procedure may be repeated several times a day. Faradization of the muscles with large, moist electrodes is also successful. Galvanization of the muscles with anode application to painful points may often be tried with good effect. In old and obstinate cases faradic massage or static sparks may be tried. *Traumatic Muscular Atrophy.*—In cases of atrophy of muscles from non-use, due to injury, diseases of the joints, or general debilitating diseases where the muscles have wasted, the faradic current, to produce strong contractions, or combined with mechanical treatment, as in farado-massage, or galvanofaradization, are useful. Local applications of static electricity (sparks and shocks) are also followed by success at times. "When the neuro-electrical irritability is preserved to either current the nutrition of the muscles can in most cases be restored. *Muscular Cicatrices and Contractures.*—In these cases the galvanic current is used for its electrolytic and trophic effects. The anode is applied to the scar, while the cathode is placed on the opposite side of the limb or moved about in a circle around the seat of the lesion, or the reverse position of the poles may be tried. Galvano-massage may be of use. *Acute Articular Rheumatism.*—R. Remak advised the application of the galvanic current stabile through the affected joints and claimed good results therefrom. More recently Drosdorff, von Beetz, Abramowski, and more particularly Lewandowski have used the faradic current with highly gratifying success. Large, moist electrodes may be used, but the favorite method of the authors mentioned is the dry faradic brush (secondary coil) applied to the skin directly over the joint until decided redness is produced. A brush may be used with either electrode, but it is customary to employ one brush and one large, moist electrode, which is applied to the limb opposite the area faradized with the brush. The current is at first weak, gradually increasing in strength. The effects are a diminution of pain, reduction of fever, shortening of the disease process, and absorption of the exudation. The sittings often require to be repeated several times a day. Lewandowski has treated seventyfive cases, with satisfactory results in all. *Chronic Articular Rheumatism.*—In these cases the electrolytic effects of the galvanic current should be brought into requisition. Strong currents should be passed directly through the joints in order to cause absorption of the effusion. The electrodes, large and well moistened, should be so placed as to get a direct permeating current. The current should be frequently reversed. Electro-massage of the joint and the surrounding structures,is of advantage in relieving pain and promoting absorption. When there is much tenderness of the joint the electric hand is indicated; in other cases the rollerelectrode (Fig. 223) may be used. General electrization, electric baths, and local faradization with the faradic brush have also been followed by success.

Fig. 223.—Roller Or Massage Electrode. *Nodular Rheumatism (Rheumatic Gout).*—This obscure and persistent affection has occasionally yielded to electricity. As the disease seems at times to have some connection with the nervous system, some electricians have performed subaural and spinal galvanization in addition to proper local electrical measures. Galvanism is used, passing the current directly through the affected joint, in order to secure the electrolytic effects. The faradic brush or moist electrodes may be employed for the relief of pain.

Articular Effusions.—In effusions into the joints, whether inflammatory or vaso-neurotic in origin, electricity is often of decided value. Transverse galvanic currents, with V. A., or faradization with the dry brush or moist electrodes, or galvanopuncture, have all been followed by success. *Traumatic Arthritis.*—The usual percutaneous, electrolytic methods, faradization with the dry brush and moist electrodes, local faradic baths, and in some cases prolonged weak galvanic currents have all been followed by success, Most non-purulent effusions into joints will yield to a rationally-conducted electrical treatment. *Hypertrophic Callus and Other Traumatic Periostoses.*— Prolonged transverse galvanization of the seat of the deposit with V. A. will often yield good results. To illustrate the importance of persistence in the treatment the following case reported by Moritz Meyer is quoted: A boy had a large, bony callus on the left arm, interfering with the motions of the elbowjoint. The flexores communis, sublimis and profundis, and the flexor longus pollicis were imbedded in the callus and their action inhibited. Meyer applied a large electrode to one surface of the arm and used a small electrode to the median nerve and then over the callus, and made numerous reversals of the current. In the course of. seven months, during which the patient had one hundred and eighteen sittings, the callus had been removed and the mobility of the joint restored. Before Meyer undertook the treatment of the case, Professor von Bergmann had examined the patient and proposed resection of the joint as the only practicable procedure. *Anchylosis, Stiffness of Joints, and Periarthritic Swellings.* — These often yield to the constant current (electrolytic current). The faradic current may sometimes aid the effect, but the principal reliance must be placed in galvanism. *Painful Neuroses of the Joints.*—The so-called joint neuralgias are readily treated by electricity. Pressure points should be searched for and subjected to the anode applications. These painful spots may usually be found in the following localities: For the spinal articulations, over the spinous processes; for the elbow, at the external condyle of the humerus and the head of the radius; for the wrist, at the styloid process of the ulna; for the hip, midway between the tuber ischii and trochanter major, a little external to the latter; for the knee, at the internal condyle, at the apex of the patella, and behind the head of the fibula; for the ankle, below each malleolus.

DISEASES OF THE EYE.

Removal of Foreign Bodies.—The removal of foreign bodies (particles of iron and steel) by means of an electromagnet has been frequently accomplished. Professor Hirschberg, of Berlin, has constructed a magnet for this purpose, with which he has operated a large number of times. In 1885 he reported thirty-three successful cases. Many modifications of this instrument have been made. One of the most convenient of these was devised by Dr. Hubbell, and is shown in Fig. 224. Dr. Hubbell claims, as advantages for this instrument, greater power of attraction, lightness, small size, shape, and convenience of manipulation.

The apparatus is connected with one cell of any kind of active battery, and the end of the magnet, projected into a fine terminal point, is placed as near as convenient to the foreign body. On closing the circuit the current passes through the wire of the electro-magnet and renders the iron core magnetic. If the foreign body is deeply imbedded in the eyeball, it may be necessary to puncture the ball and insert the point of the electromagnet until the foreign particle can be attracted by it and removed. The battery circuit must not be broken until the particle is entirely removed from the eye. By means of this instrument particles of iron have been removed from the vitreous humor without adding to the injury already sustained by the organ.

Angiomata of the lids may be readily destroyed by electrolysis. A needle-electrode (Fig. 225) is used as cathode and moderate destruction of the morbid growth produced, especial attention being directed to the enlarged vessels, obliteration of which must be attempted. If a current of proper strength is employed, the tissues around the needle become pale, then grayish and puffy from the infiltration of gas. There is usually no bleeding on withdrawal of the needle, but should any follow it can be easily arrested by reversing the current, making the

Fig. 225.—Needle-Electrode. needle positive and re-inserting it. This produces a firm clot and arrests all bleeding promptly. The positive electrode should be the ordinary sponge or cotton-covered electrode, which may be applied to'the temple or on an indifferent point. It is usually most convenient to apply it to the back of the hand. The needle should be of gold or platinum in order to avoid corrosion. A steel needle will not be attacked by the fluids around the negative pole, but it is difficult to prevent its oxidation, while if it is required to use it as the anode it is quickly corroded by the fluids set free around the positive pole, and then becomes difficult to remove without producing a good deal of disturbance of the clot or tissues. In some cases, also, the black oxide of iron formed may remain as a permanent tattoomark.

Great care should be taken not to produce too much destruction at one time, for a large slough may leave a disfiguring scar. If the electrolysis is performed carefully the result will be very satisfactory. The most important requisite for a good result is patience.

Small areas (about one square centimetre) should be taken at a sitting. With the electrodes mentioned, a current of 2 to 3 milliamperes is adequate to produce sufficient destruction. The needle may be kept in one position four or five minutes and then carefully withdrawn and re-inserted at a little distance. The circuit should be broken before withdrawing the needle.

Other new growths, such as papillomata, pigmentary naevi, and even epitheliomata, are destroyed with nearly equal readiness by means of electrolysis. The needle is used as cathode, the anode being placed on any convenient portion of the body. A current of from 1 to 4 milliamperes is used for four or five minutes at a time, the base of the growth being perforated in several directions with the needle. The destroyed growth shrivels up and drops off in the course of a week or ten days, leaving a dry, brownish spot, which gradually fades to white. The only dressing required is an application of hot water once or twice a day, for four or five minutes, and repeated on two or three successive days.

The galvano-cautery knife or snare can also be used for the destruction of small growths about the eyelids.

In Trichiasis, so difficult to cure by any other method, brilliant results are obtained with electrolysis. In fact, the present extensive employment of electrolysis in dermatology dates from its use by Dr. Michel, of St. Louis, in treating trichiasis. The cathodic needle is used with a current of to 2 milliamperes, the sensibility of the lids having first been obtunded with a 10-per-cent. solution of cocaine. The cathodic needle is carefully inserted into the follicle of the misdirected lash, and the circuit closed, either with the contact closer in the handle, or with the anode. The current is passed until the hair can be removed without resistance by means of a pair of epilating forceps. Then the circuit is broken and the needle withdrawn. If the operation has been carefully performed the hair thus removed will not grow again. *Inflammation of the Meibomian Follicles and Chalazion* may also be successfully treated by electrolysis. The needle, a cathode, is inserted into the small swelling, and a mild current passed a few minutes. A channel remains through which the contents, purulent or cheesy, may discharge. The walls of the little cysts in chalazion are also stimulated to healthy action, and recovery follows. *Entropion and Ectropion* have been treated successfully by long-continued faradization of the orbicularis palpebrarum muscle, using fine electrodes. In entropion, however, the galvano-cautery will produce quicker results if a small strip of skin is deeply seared and allowed to heal by cicatrization. The contraction of the linear cicatrix turns the border of the lids outward. *Spasms of the Eyelids* are treated with mild galvanic currents, applying the anode to painful spots, if any are present. Galvanization of the medulla oblongata and subaural galvanization are also employed. Anode application to the closed lids. cathode indifferent, has been tried with good effect. Swelling faradic currents (Far. » and V. A. have been used. Lewandowski relates a case of reflex blepharospasm, in which the spasm of the orbicularis and corrugator followed ten days after a sabre-cut of the left cheek. The spasms were severe and constant. A single sitting, with galvanization of the medulla oblongata, anode to back of neck, cathode in the hand, relieved the spasm perfectly. Spasms of the ocular muscles are treated on the same principles as other facial spasms *(q. v.).*

Trachoma is sometimes treated by electrolysis. The double electrode (Fig. 226) is a convenient method of producing absorption or thinning of the abnormally thickened mucous membrane.

Paralyses of Ocular Muscles.—These may be of central but are mostly of peripheral (rheumatic, syphilitic, diphtheritic) origin. The prognosis is usually favorable in recent cases. The electrical treatment is partly directed to the centres (brain galvanization), and partly to the paralyzed nerves and muscles. The cathode may be applied over the closed eyelids, and the anode to the back of the neck or the occipital region of the opposite side. If the conjunctiva is anaesthetized with cocaine the muscles can be directly stimulated with a fine electrode (Ca.) through the conjunctival sac, as practiced by Gozzini and M. Rosenthal, the anode being applied over the forehead. Peripheral faradization or galvano-faradization may also be tried. Subaural galvanization is sometimes useful. Soetlin has successfully treated acquired nystagmus with galvanization of the eyeball, a large electrode (Ca.) being applied over the closed eye, and the anode placed upon an indifferent point. Short sittings (one-half to one and one-half minutes) are indicated. *Mydriasis.*—The anode may be placed over the closed eye, and the cathode swept around the orbit. Direct faradization of the eyeball, after cocainization, may also be tried. *Muscular Asthenopia* may sometimes be cured by galvanization of the internal rectus. The cathode is applied over the inner angle of the closed eyelids. *Corneal Affections.*—Keratitis of various kinds has frequently been treated successfully with electricity. In phlyctenular keratitis faradization of the conjunctiva, with a moist camel'shair pencil as an electrode, has been used, or one electrode may be applied over the closed eyelids, and the other in the nape of the neck. The galvanic current may also be used, and success has been reported with it in neuroparalytic ophthalmia and parenchymatous keratitis. Subaural galvanization has been employed in pannous keratitis. Opacities of the cornea have been successfully treated by means of electrolysis, and special electrodes have been devised for this purpose. Adler proceeds in the following manner: A small, moistened metal plate (anode).. is applied to the scleral conjunctiva, and the cathode, a small silver spatula, is passed with slight pressure over the opacity. A current of 1 to 1 milliamperes is employed, and the sitting continued for only ten to twenty seconds. Atropia is then instilled, and the eye bandaged. In a few days the signs of irritation disappear, and much improvement is manifested in the appearance and usefulness of the eye.

The galvano-cautery has also been used with excellent results in corneal affections. In rapidly-destructive or infective ulcerations, the prompt use of the galvano-cautery will often save the organ from destruction.

Diseases of the Iris.—In iritis, the electrolytic current through a large moist electrode over the closed lids has been used successfully. Hypopion has also been successfully treated by means of direct faradization, a fine sponge electrode being applied to the lower border of the cornea, and the region of the purulent collection being touched three or four times during the sitting. *Diseases of the Choroid.*—Chronic inflammatory affections of the choroid, with pigment deposits, plastic exudations, or atrophic spots are favorably influenced by the galvanic current. One electrode is placed upon the brow and the other behind the ear of the same side. *Diseases of the Lens.*—Opacities of the lens from various causes have been subjected to the galvanic current with asserted success. Giraud-Teulon states that electricity is the mostt effective and rapid method of treatment of all forms of cloudiness of the lens. Whether it is equally effective in true cataract is doubtful, although Neftel has reported good results.

The galvanic current is used. The electrodes are applied so as to secure direct transmission of the current through the eyeball. One electrode may be applied over the closed eye and the other to the back of the neck, the mastoid process, or the subaural fossa. The current should be passed alternately in both directions. Weak currents and short sittings, three to five minutes, should be the rule.

Diseases of the Retina.—Atrophy of the optic nerve, either primary or in the course of posterior spinal sclerosis, may sometimes be improved by the proper and persistent use of galvanism, but the prospect is not very encouraging. A number of cases are reported, however, and, in the absence of any other trustworthy treatment of this affection at our command, electricity should be given a patient trial. In optic neuritis and secondary atrophy, the results are usually more favorable. Decided improvement can often be obtained, and in a considerable number of cases the functional activity of the eye may again approach the normal standard. *Amblyopia and Amaurosis,* consequent upon toxic causes, hysterical visual abnormalities, and other disturbances of vision, for which no anatomical lesions can be found, are all more or less favorable conditions for electrical treatment. The methods are: Transverse frontal galvanization; galvanization from the closed eyelids to the mastoid process, or nape of the neck; subaural galvanization, galvano-faradization, and the dry galvanic brush, according to Rumpf's method. The results in most cases depend upon electrolytic and reflex trophic effects of currents. *Stricture of the Nasal Duct* should yield with especial facility to electrolysis properly applied,—cathode in the duct by means of an insulated sound, anode in the palm of the hand. Weekly sittings. Trial should be made of the method.

DISEASES OF THE EAR.

Noises in the Ear, Hyperesthesias, Parcesthesias, and Torpor of the Auditory Nerve are all more or less susceptible to improvement by electrical treatment. Brenner, who developed to such a high degree the physiological reactions of the auditory apparatus to the electric current (see p. 155), also contributed much to our knowledge of the therapeutic application of electricity in aural affections. The galvanic current is usually employed, although faradization and static electricity have been used very successfully by some practitioners. *Tinnitus Aurium,* depending upon nervous disorders, has been treated by transverse or diagonal brain galvanization,— from mastoid to mastoid, or from mastoid of one side to the back of the neck of the other side. Good results have been obtained in some cases by these methods. The "polar method" of Brenner is, however, generally adopted. This is based upon the physiological reactions to the galvanic current. If there is electrical hyperesthesia of the auditory nerve, the normal sound sensations produced by opening and closing of the current with the different poles arc simply intensified. This may be present with tinnitus. The normal formula of sound reactions may also be reversed. In this case the character of the reaction furnishes an indication for the treatment. Thus, in a case of tinnitus let the anode first be employed, placing the cathode at an indifferent point, as the palm of the hand. If the noises are not modified, or are even increased, the other pole is tried. The anode-closing and anode-duration reactions are first tested, and if they produce no abatement, or an increase in the noises, the pole is reversed and the cathodic reactions tested. Brenner, Erb, Hagen, and Moos have reported cases in which treatment based upon the galvanic acoustic reaction was followed by prompt relief. In the majority of cases the anode treatment was successful. When a modification or disappearance of the noises has been obtained, the current should be gradually diminished with the rheostat in order to avoid the sudden shock when the current is broken. The current used should not be strong enough to produce vertigo. In nervous deafness pretty strong currents with V. A. are sometimes necessary to obtain any reaction. The active electrode is usually applied directly over the ear, or upon the mastoid process, but sometimes a special aural electrode, insulated by a rubber speculum-tube (Fig. 227), is inserted into the external auditory meatus, which is filled with warm water. In this way the current is more strictly localized, but no special superiority in results over the external application of the electrode has been observed. The external application of the faradic current has also been followed by success, while Benedict claims brilliant results with static electricity, drawing a fine spray of sparks from the drum membrane. *Nervous Deafness* unaccompanied by tinnitus may also at times be successfully treated by the galvanic current. The same methods of application are employed.

In bilateral affections of the auditory nerve it is often useful to have the active electrode double; that is to say, a double conducting cord for the pole which is applied to the ear (Fig. 228). In this way both ears are treated at the same time.

Fig. 227.—Aural ElecTrode. *Deficient Secretion of Cerumen.*—The galvanic current is often useful in this annoying condition. The meatus is filled with warm water, the insulated ear-electrode introduced and connected with the negative pole. The anode may be applied over the mastoid process, or held in the hand. The secretion soon becomes freer and the pliability of the lining membrane of the canal restored. It is probable that chronic inflammation and thickening of the membrane, or stenosis, would also yield to appropriate electrical treatment.

Thickening and opacity of the tympanic membrane may be treated by the galvanic current, the cathode being placed in the meatus, filled with warm water, and the anode applied to the mastoid process, the back of the neck, or held in the hand.

Polypi in the external meatus may be destroyed by electrolysis, the pedicle being transfixed with the cathode-needle electrode, and a weak current passed. The galvano-cautery is, however, more prompt in its effects, and little, if any, more painful.

Chronic Middle-Ear Catarrh.—It is the prevalent opinion among otologists that most cases of deafness depend upon chronic inflammatory conditions of the tympanic cavity, associated with chronic catarrh and collapse or stenosis of the Eustachian tube. Weber-Liel has highly recommended the application of electricity to tone up the relaxed walls of the tube in these cases. He states that in the first stage of the disease, when the muscu

Fig. 229.—Electrode For Eustachian Tdbe. lar walls of the tube still react to the electrical stimulus, electricity is indicated. The effects are especially marked in young persons, and after two or more sittings the hearing is often greatly improved. The subjective aural symptoms (noises, etc.) may still continue, but will also yield to a continuance of the treatment. Only in the later stages, when the atrophic changes in the muscles of the tube and of the ossicles have progressed so far that the electrical reaction is entirely destroyed, no improvement is to be expected. The sittings may sometimes require to be extended to fifteen or twenty minutes. The active electrode (Ca.), in the form of a fine-wire stilet, is inserted into the tube through a rubber catheter (Fig. 229), and the other electrode may be applied over the ear or along the cervical spine. It is strange that in an affection so little amenable to treatment by other methods more numerous observations have not been made by specialists in aural diseases, especially as the conditions seem particularly favorable for obtaining good results from electrical treatment.

DISEASES OF THE NOSE.

The functional disturbances of the sense of smell may sometimes be relieved by galvanization of the Schneiderian mucous membrane, but a more numerous class of diseases of

Fig. 230.—Nasal Electrode. the nose are susceptible to electrolytic treatment. Hartmann has recently recorded his favorable experience with the galvanic current in hypertrophic rhinitis, and Voltolini has removed nasal polypi by means of electrolysis. In the case of polypi and other tumors of the nasal cavity, however, the galvano-cautery offers such excellent advantages that it is unlikely to be replaced by any of the slower and perhaps less efficient measures. Fig. 230 shows an electrode used in hypertrophic catarrh.

DISEASES OF THE TONGUE.

Ulcers, paretic conditions, and new growths may require electrical treatment to produce desired improvement. Functional disorders of the sense of taste so frequently depend upon brain-lesions that their treatment is to be referred to the latter. Ulcers and new formations may be subjected to electrolytic treatment or to the more rapidly acting galvano-cautery. A slight cauterization of a lingual ulcer with the galvano-cautery will often cause the healing of the ulcer and prevent development of a cancer. Fig. 231 shows an electrode for treating ulcers of the tongue by electrolysis, or for electrical stimulation of the muscular substance of the organ.

DISEASES OF THE RESPIRATORY ORGANS.

Aphasia, Aphonia, and Aphthongia.—Cases of these affections often yield with' surprising promptness to electricity. The effects are largely dependent upon the cause. When the affection is hysterical, intra-pharyngeal or transverse laryngeal faradization are usually successful. Galvanization of the spine is also sometimes useful. When aphasia is due to an anatomical lesion of the speech-centre, longitudinal, transverse, and diagonal brain galvanization are indicated. When loss of speech is caused by intra-laryngeal growths the galvano-cautery snare or electrolysis under cocaine will be appropriate measures of treatment. A papillomatous growth of the vocal cord can be readily removed by either method. *Hysterical Paraesthesias of the Throat and Larynx.*—Transverse laryngeal galvanization or faradization are effective in many cases. The dry faradic brush may also be used to the front of the neck. Galvanism to the cervical spine, or from the spine to the larynx, may be tried in some cases with hope of success. *Nervous Asthma.* —This is often treated with success by electricity. Some practitioners use the galvanic current, others find better results follow faradization. Subaural and pneumogastric galvanization—anode to the back of the neck, cathode between larynx and sterno-cleido-mastoid muscle—have been very successfully used by Brenner and Neftel. Spinal galvanization from the cervical to the lumbar spine have yielded good results in some cases. Transverse faradization of the chest with strong currents may be useful. *Asphyxia.*—When due to inhalations of poisonous gases or vapors, or the ingestion of poisons, or to arrest of respiration in other ways (asphyxia neonatorum, diphtheria), this has been treated successfully with the electric current. The method employed is that of faradization of the phrenic nerves. Either of two procedures may be adopted: (1) both electrodes are placed over the motor points for the phrenic nerves in the neck (see Fig. 138, page 162); or (2) one electrode is placed over one phrenic nerve, and the other applied over the pit of the stomach. The current should be interrupted once every three seconds, in order to promote rhythmical contractions of the diaphragm.

DISEASES OF THE ORGANS OF CIRCULATION.

Angina Pectoris.—During the attacks cutaneous faradization with the dry brush over the cardiac region, as recommended by Duchenne, may be tried. This method cuts short the attack. Direct faradization of the cardiac region, using large, moist electrodes and strong currents from spine to front of thorax, has also been successfully employed. Eulenbnrg uses galvanism, cathode to the spine, anode over the heart. Subaural and vagus galvanization and galvanization of the cervical portion of the cord should be persistently followed up during the intervals. Static electricity has also been used with success in the forms of static breeze and insulation. *Dilatation of the Heart.*—Von Ziemssen has recommended the transverse galvanization of the dilated and weak heart as a means of strengthening the same. The current is passed from the spine to the cardiac region. Experiments by Herbst and Dixon Mann render it doubtful whether any direct effect can be produced upon the heart by this method of using the current, but the final appeal must be to clinical experience. The careful observation of appropriate cases subjected to electrical treatment will demonstrate the usefulness or otherwise of this procedure. *Aneurism.* —"When a galvanic current is passed through blood or other liquid containing albumen, the latter is coagulated. The coagulation takes place at both electrodes, if both are immersed in the albuminous fluid, but the clot around the anode is much denser than that around the cathode.

These phenomena of the galvanic current led to the trial of this agent in the treatment of aneurisms situated in regions of the body or upon vessels not accessible to the ligature, compression, or other means of surgical treatment. The first physician who attempted the cure of aneurism by electricity was Petrequin. of Lyons, who operated upon his first case in 1845. After him Ciniselli, Robin, Dujardin-Beaumetz, and others employed thb treatment with more or less success. Up to the present time considerably more than one hundred cases have been so treated, and probably one-fourth of the number may be said to have been cured, or the symptoms much alleviated. Dangerous results from the operation itself are rare, and, where proper care is used, are not likely to occur. It is reasonable to suppose that the many failures in the earlier reports of cases treated are due to improper methods employed, and perhaps also to the fact that generally only otherwise hopeless cases are selected for trial of a new method of treatment.

The effects of galvano-puncture of aneurism are due to electrolysis. The current decomposes the blood, and by recombination of chemical elements at the electrodes—the so-called "secondary" electrolysis—coagulation of albumen compound takes place. The phenomena of electrolysis, already described (page 255), can here be readily recognized. If both pole (armed with needles), be plunged into the tumor, the clot around the positive is firm and dense, that around the negative soft and permeated with small bubbles of (hydrogen) gas.

In the earlier operations for galvanopuncture (or, more properly, electrolysis) of aneurism, both poles were introduced into the tumor. The consequence was that two kinds of clot were produced, one of which (the soft cathodic clot) had a strong tendency to break down and soften. Some bad results were thus produced.

In more recent trials, however, the anode alone was introduced into the aneurismal sac, the cathode being applied externally. In this way but one sort of clot, a firm one, was produced, which adhered to the sides of the sac, and showed little tendency to break down or become detached and form dangerous embolisms. The perfected method of introducing but one pole (the anode) into the sac, and carefully regulating the current used with a rheostat and milliamperemeter, deserves

Fig. 232.—Needle-electrode For Electrolysis Of Aneurism. to be more extensively tried in a malady which offers such slight prospects of cure with any other method of treatment.

The method of employing electrolysis in aneurism is as follows:—

One or more gold or platinum needles, insulated to within one inch of the point, in order to avoid action on the skin and other tissues intervening between the surface and the sac, are plunged into the sac to a sufficient depth to entirely immerse the uninsulated portions in the fluid contents of the tumor. The other ends of the needles, if more than one be used, are then connected with a conducting cord by means of a collecting contact (shown in Fig. 232). The needles are connected with the positive pole of the battery.

As the negative pole a large electrode, either of carbon, clay, or metal, covered with moist absorbent cotton, is used. Wire-gauze sheets make very convenient electrodes (Fig. 233).

They are flexible, and can easily be made to fit snugly any surface. They should be covered with a moist layer of absorbent cotton. A bath-towel well moistened with salt solution answers the purpose very well.

The negative electrode is first applied where it will not be in the way. If the aneurism is thoracic, the electrode may be applied over the abdomen, and *vice versâ*. After making sure of all contacts and the proper working condition of the battery, the needles are then successively plunged into the aneurismal sac. With the milliamperemeter in the circuit, the cells are then gradually added, one by one, until a current of 20 to 30 milliamperes is shown by the meter. This may be allowed to act for ten minutes and then the current is gradually reduced by dropping out of circuit the cells one at a time. If there is a good rheostat in the circuit, this should be used to increase and diminish the strength of the current. If it be attempted now to withdraw the needles from the sac, it will be found that they are pretty firmly fixed in their positions. This is owing to the closeness and density of the clot. Should they be removed by forcibly pulling upon them, the clot may be disturbed in position and allow bleeding from the interior of the sac through the puncture, or portions of the clot may be broken off and be washed along in the blood-current, and cause embolism. For this reason the needles should be first gently rotated to loosen them from the coagulum and very gradually withdrawn. A better method is, however, after diminishing the current to zero, to reverse the poles making the needles negative, and then sending a moderate current through the circuit in the opposite direction for a minute or two. This produces a little disintegration immediately around the needles, and they can then be removed, not only without force, but without danger of causing haemorrhage.

After withdrawal of the needles the punctures are covered with a little antiseptic cotton and painted over with collodion. It goes without saying, that strict antiseptic precautions should be observed throughout the operation. The needles must be disinfected and the skin thoroughly washed with a disinfectant solution of mercuric bichloride. It will hardly be necessary to add that the operator's hands should likewise be in an aseptic condition.

After the operation the patient should be kept quiet for several days. If symptoms of inflammation manifest themselves they should be combated by hot or cold applications and such other measures as are rationally indicated.

Sometimes a single sitting is sufficient to produce coagulation of the entire mass of blood in the sac. In others, a number are required. In this event, the sittings may be repeated every ten to fifteen days. Anaesthetics are rarely, if ever, necessary.

DISEASES OF THE ABDOMINAL ORGANS.

The galvanic, faradic, or combined currents passed through the abdominal walls cause contraction of the muscular coats of the stomach and intestines, and may in this way act favorably in torpidity of the gastro-intestinal tract, dilatation of the stomach, chronic constipation, etc., or even, by producing regular vermicular movements, may cause restoration of displaced gut in invagination or hernia.

Neuroses of the Stomach and Intestines.—Gastralgia, enteralgia, and colic often yield to the galvanic current. The anode (large, moist electrode) is placed over the seat of pain, and the cathode over the spine, or an indifferent point. Strong currents may be required to arrest the pain. Central and subaural galvanization are sometimes useful, especially in gastralgia. Energetic applications of fnradism by means of the dry faradic brush over the epigastrium are often effectual.

The treatment should be persisted in during the intervals of the attacks. Daily sittings of ten minutes' duration, using weak currents gradually increased and decreased, or swelling faradization may be employed.

Nervous Heart-burn and Nervous Dyspepsia.—Most practitioners now recognize a form of dyspepsia, not dependent upon structural lesions of the stomach, or tangible dietetic error. This, whether considered merely as a symptom of general neurasthenia, or as an individual affection, none the less often requires individual treatment. In these cases, in addition to regimenal measures, electricity is often of great service. The galvanic current employed in the forms of central, subaural, and vertebro-epigastric galvanization; transverse faradization and faradic baths, or static electricity in the forms of insulation and static breeze are all indicated.

Intestinal "nervous dyspepsia" acpompanied by flatulence, enteralgia, frequent diarrhoeas, etc., should be treated upon the same principles and by similar methods.

Nervous (Reflex) Vomiting—Vomiting of Pregnancy.—In this often troublesome symptom the application of electricity will often bring about a prompt cessation of the vomiting. The methods are galvanization or faradization from the cervical spine to the epigastrium. Both poles of the faradic battery may also be placed over the right and left hypochondriac regions, and the current passed from side to side. Mild currents from the cervix uteri to the spine have also been used. In addition to these local applications, subaural or vagus galvanization may be used. *Atony and Dilatation of the Stomach.*—In the treatment of this condition von Ziemssen has reported most encouraging results, confirming those of Onimus, Neftel, De Watteville, and others. Large electrodes are employed, one being placed over the left hypochondriac region, somewhat posteriorly, and the other in the epigastrium. Strong faradic currents, frequently interrupted, or galvano-faradization should be employed. Daily sittings of five to ten minutes are recommended. Other measures for the relief of the same condition (lavage, dietetic regulation) should be combined with the electrical treatment. Galvanism, employed in the same way as faradism, has also been used with success. Some practitioners use an intra-gastric electrode, applying the other over the region of the stomach externally, but it is doubtful whether much better results are obtained than when the percutaneous method is employed. If the internal method is employed, the stomach should first be filled with water to promote the diffusion of the current and prevent too intense irritation of the portions of the mucous membrane touched by the electrode. *Intestinal Obstruction.*—When this is due to atony, or paralysis of the intestinal walls, electricity is the rationally indicated remedy. Galvanization, faradization, or galvano-faradization may be used. The usual method is to insert one electrode into the rectum and apply the other labile over the course of the colon. The faradic current is usually employed, although galvanization, with voltaic alternatives has also given successful results. When the galvanic current is used, care must be taken to prevent electrolytic action by the rectal electrode. Lead colic yields to the same methods of application of electricity.

In intestinal obstruction following invagination, electricity has likewise been used with marked success. Various methods are employed, most of them being similar to those mentioned in

Pig. 234.—Boudet's Intestinal Electrode. the preceding paragraph. Dr. Boudet, of Paris, has devised an intestinal catheter-electrode, which has been used with success by himself, Rapin, and others. It is shown in Fig. 234. *M* is an insulated catheter with an exposed tip, *S*. This is connected with the negative pole of the battery by means of a contact screw shown at *C*. *T* is a rubber tube through which salt solution can be injected or infused into the intestine. The instrument is inserted well up into the intestinal canal, and about a quart of warm salt water forced into the gut. The anode consists of a large electrode about five inches square, which is applied to the back. A current of 10 to 50 milliamperes is used from five to ten minutes. The current may be reversed or interrupted at intervals. The faradic current may likewise be used by this method.

Habitual Constipation.—This troublesome and frequent disorder yields in many cases to the proper employment of electricity. The methods of application vary, and success has been obtained with all. Both electrodes may be applied to the abdominal walls and moved about in a way to make the current pass through the abdominal cavity and its contents. When the galvanic current is employed, the anode may be applied over the spine, and the cathode moved over the abdomen along the course of the colon. The current may frequently be reversed or interrupted. In obstinate cases, Erb follows the galvanic application with faradization. Both currents may be combined after the manner of De Watteville. The apparatus of Boudet, shown on preceding page, may also be used in constipation. In most cases a rectal electrode, combined with abdominal faradization, will give very good results. The sittings should be repeated daily. Improvement in the tone of the intestinal walls is gradual, but rarely fails to follow the proper use of the remedy. *Prolapsus Ani.*—This condition has been repeatedly treated with success by the various methods of local electrization. Galvanic, or faradic, or combined currents from the spine or abdomen to the rectum, or from the sacrum to the perinaeum, have proven curative. The faradic current is the rationally indicated one. *Stricture of the Rectum.*—The cure of stricture of the rectum by means of electrolysis has been the subject of considerable discussion among surgeons. A number of cases of successful operation has been reported by competent observers, and the procedure may be regarded as an established one in surgery. In a paper read before the American Medical Association in 1889, Dr Robert Newman reviews the whole question, and gives a history of all reported cases. The strictures most amenable to electrolysis are the infiltrated ones so frequently the result of late.syphilitic lesions, and which are not readily amenable to any other safe method of treatment. The electrolytic method is safe, comparatively painless, and infinitely less tedious than the ordinary method of dilatation with flexible bougies.

In treating a case of rectal stricture with electrolysis, the size of the stricture should be first carefully measured by means of bulbous sounds, or, in default of a better instrument, with Otis' urethrameter. Electrodes of proper size and shape (Fig. 235) should be procured, and at the first sitting one a few millimetres larger than the lumen of the stricture should be employed. The electrode should be attached as cathode, placing the anode in the form of a large cotton-covered plate electrode upon the thigh or sacrum. A current of from 5 to 20 milliamperes may be employed, and the sittings last from five to ten minutes. The rectum should first be washed out with an antiseptic solution, and if the strictured portion is very sensitive a solution of cocaine may be thrown in before beginning the sitting. If the electrode has been properly selected and the strict ure is amenable to electrolytic treatment, the sound will usually pass the strictured portion of the gut within five minutes. The patient may take a hot sitz-bath after the operation, but no other application need be made. There is sometimes some irritation and soreness in the rectum, particularly if the stronger currents have been employed. Sittings may be repeated weekly unless the reaction is severe. The size of the electrode must be gradually increased as the strictured portion of the gut is widened, but patience is the first of virtues here, for if attempts are made to dilate too rapidly, either by increasing the size of the sounds, decreasing the intervals between sittings, or using too strong currents, failure or disappointment are likely to result.

Haemorrhoids.—The coagulating property of the positive pole makes the electrolytic current a valuable means of treating haemorrhoids. While not as prompt or effective as the clamp and cautery method of ablation, electrolysis gives much more promise of success than the various methods of injection of coagulating or irritant substances, such as carbolic acid, ergot, iodine, tincture of chloride of iron, etc. The positive electrode, armed with a needle, should be used, the cathode consisting of a large, moist plate-electrode applied to the buttock or sacrum. The current may be from ten to twenty milliamperes. The cathode is first applied to the desired surface, and fixed in position; then the needle is inserted in one of the tumors and the current gradually increased to the desired strength. The current should be allowed to pass until all the blood in the hemorrhoid is solidified, when the current is decreased to zero, reversed, and allowed to pass for a minute or two in order to loosen the needle. Steel needles are not applicable, those made of gold or platinum being the best, as they are not attacked by the fluids around the positive pole. Each separate pile should be thus attacked and its contents solidified. This need not be done at one sitting, but may be divided among several sittings at intervals of a week. Swelling, pain, or inflammation may be combated by hot-water applications. The after-treatment must be conducted on general antiseptic principles. *Portal Congestion.*—Galvano-faradization of the right hypochondriac region gives some promise of success. *Catarrhal Jaundice.*—When the trouble is obstinate, faradization of the gall-bladder, or rather of the abdominal wall above the gall-bladder, may be useful. Gerhardt has reported a case in which all other measures tried failed to relieve, but which yielded to abdominal faradization. The explanation given is that the compression of the gall-bladder by the contracting abdominal muscles forced a way for the bile through the common duct. *Enlargement of the Spleen.*—The enlargement of the spleen following chronic malarial poisoning and typhoid lever yields in the happiest manner to faradization. The methods used are either percutaneous faradization, with large, moist electrodes over the splenic region, or the dry faradic brush applied to the abdominal walls. In the latter method each electrode is armed with a brush. The sittings are repeated daily and last about three minutes. The decrease in size of the splenic tumor is measurable by percussion, and is said to be permanent. Chvostek and Lewandowski report success in from 75 to 80 per cent, of the cases treated. *Ascites.*—Abdominal dropsy from whatever cause may often be temporarily caused to disappear by electricity. Most observers who have treated ascites by this agent have employed the faradic current. The secretion of urine is increased and the dropsy rapidly disappears. Where the effusion is due to structural diseases of the liver, heart, or kidneys, permanency of the effect cannot, of course, be expected. The galvanic current should *a priori* offer even better results. *Diabetes Mellitus and Insipidus.*—Several cases have been reported in which beneficial effects have followed the application of electricity in these diseases. Neftel, Beard, and he Fort have seen marked improvement in diabetes mellitus, following subaural and spinal galvanization. Central galvanization would seem rationally indicated. Ranney has seen improvement follow static insulation in similar cases.

In diabetes insipidus successful cases are reported in considerable number. Galvanization and faradization of the renal region has been used with success. Erb advises central and subaural galvanization and general faradization, in addition to the local application of the current.

DISEASES OF THE FEMALE GENERATIVE APPARATUS.

At the present time the use of electricity in the diseases of women is one of the great medical questions of the day. Although this agent has been employed for many years in the treatment of female sexual disorders and in obstetrics, it is mainly due to the labors of Dr. George Apostoli, of Paris, that the question has assumed its present commanding position. While Tripier, Althaus, Cutter, Neftel, Dixon Mann, Beard, and Rockwell preceded Apostoli, and "blazed the way," as it were, the latter is regarded, and with justice, as the creator of the art of scientifically applying electricity in diseases of the female pelvic viscera.

The remarkable results reported by Apostoli as having followed the use of strong galvanic currents (100 to 250 ma.) in uterine fibroids were at first received with incredulity by gynaecologists. However, the adhesion of Sir Spencer Wells and Dr. Thomas Keith, unquestionably the foremost gynaecological surgeons living, to Apostoli's views and methods of treatment have placed the latter upon a plane where they demand the attention of all progressive practitioners.

And this attention is not withheld. In the United States and Great Britain the gynaecologists seem to be divided into two hostile forces, one having faith in the power of the electric current to correct many of the morbid conditions of the female sexual organs, while the other denies all virtue to this remedy, or allows it standing merely in the relief of certain "functional" difficulties. It is worthy of remark, however, that in general the adherents of the electrical treatment are those who have studied and made personal trial of it, while its opponents and contemners are men who have never investigated it fairly, or who consider it beneath the dignity of a "surgeon" to meddle with such gewgaws as batteries, electrodes, and milliamperemeters. The intelligent and thinking reader will be able to determine without difficulty which of these two classes is entitled to the greater credit.

The electrical current is used in one or other of its forms in most of the diseases peculiar to women. In some affections it is still employed empirically, as it is in the diseases of the nervous system and other organs. In some, however, the indications have been rationally formulated, and precise directions for the kind of current and manner of application have been laid down.

Amenorrhaea.—As is well known, this may be due to entire absence, defective development, or temporary pathological condition of the organs necessary to the production and excretion of the menses. In the first case electrical treatment will be of as little avail as any other method, but in the second and third much benefit may be expected from the proper employment of electricity. Both galvanic and faradic currents are useful, and static electricity has been employed with success.

The methods of application are, for the faradic current, general faradization, dorso-abdominal faradization, and the dry brush to the abdominal walls, the insides of the thighs, or the soles of the feet.

When galvanism is used, central and subaural galvanization, galvanization of the spine, currents from the lumbar region to the pubis, and intra-uterine negative galvanization are the methods employed.

Although it is probably more effective to apply the electricity to the uterus, either directly or through the abdominal 'walls, electro-therapeutists generally agree that electricity applied to a distant part of the body increases the menstrual flow, or may stimulate it when it has been arrested. Hence, central and subaural galvanization are often all that is required to restore the menstrual function, if the arrest is not due to a physiological cause (pregnancy).

Dysmenorrhoea.—The books describe four or five different classes of dysmenorrhoea. The electrical treatment is more or less effective in all, but modifications in the methods of application are necessary to secure the best results. It will be advisable to consider the different kinds of the affection separately.

Obstructive Dysmenorrhoea.—When this is due to stenosis of the cervix, the galvanic current, with the cathode in the cervix, is indicated. A large, well-moistened electrode (about fifty square inches) is applied as anode over the abdomen. The current strength employed may vary from 10 to 30 milliamperes. Sittings should last ten minutes, or until the electrode passes the constriction. The electrode is an insulated sound, shown in Fig. 236, and fitted with tips of different sizes.

Sittings should begin about a week after the menstrual period, and be repeated once or twice a week until a patulous canal is secured. Occasional sittings should be had in the intervals between successive periods in order to maintain the patency of the cervix.

II 14 17 SO I——M6B«gfiailM«H—WW—i

Fig. 238.—Dk. Fry's Intra-uterine Electrode For Stenosis.

Dr. T. A. Ashby, of Baltimore, claims that the anode used in a similar manner gives equally good results. The general opinion among gynaecologists who have tried electrolysis for cervical stenosis is that it is far superior in its action to forcible dilatation with tents or steel dilators, or discission of the os.

Acute flexion of the uterus is also often a cause of obstructive dysmenorrhcea. In these cases electricity is used in the. same manner as for stenosis. The uterus is gradually straightened out, and if the treatment is continued sufficiently long the weakened segment of the uterus at the point of flexion seems

Fig. 237.—Apostolus Bipolar Intra-uterin« Electrode For Faradic Current. to become strengthened, and the normal position of the organ is maintained without other support. . Massey reports a case of sharp anteflexion cured after four sittings. Tbe positive pole was used in the uterus, and strong currents (35 to 80 milliamperes) applied for two to three minutes.

Apostoli uses in the same condition faradization with a bipolar electrode. The current of the secondary spiral (" current Electricity in the Diseases of Women, p. 12. Philadelphia, 1889. of tension ") is employed by him. By the use of this electrode (Fig. 237) Apostoli claims that the current is not dispersed, but limited to the uterus and surrounding tissues, just where its effects are desired. As this faradic current has no electrolytic or cauterizing action its strength is entirely regulated by the sensations of the patient. Sittings of from five to twenty minutes are proper. Lumbo-abdominal faradization has also been successfully employed. *Congestive Dysmenorrhea.*—In this form of painful menstruation the faradic current, either intra-uterine (Apostoli's method), or from the lumbar spine to the cervix, or dry faradic brush over the abdomen, or galvanism from the cervix to the abdomen or spine may be used. Anode to cervix, cathode externally. When galvanization is employed, weak currents and short sittings daily should be the rule.

Fig. 238.—Apostoli's Bipolar Vaginal Electrode For Faradic Current.

I *Ovarian or Nervous Dysmenorrlioea.*—In the cases where the pain is particularly localized in the ovarian region, and is unaccompanied by febrile disturbance or other evidence of inflammation, the faradic current, according to the method of Apostoli, either intra-uterine or vaginal, may usually be relied on. Where the intra-uterine electrode cannot for any reason be employed, a similar bipolar vaginal electrode (Fig. 238) is used.

The anode treatment of painful ovaries or local static electrization in the form of sparks may also be employed. The galvanic current may be localized in the neighborhood of the ovaries by using Munde's ovarain ball-electrode. The current may also be used externally to both ovarian regions by using Murray's double ovarian electrode (Fig. 239).

Membranous Dysmenorrlioea.—This may be regarded as one form of obstructive dysmenorrhcea, but the treatment most applicable is active intra-uterine "chemical cauterization," as advised by Apostoli for endometritis.

Non-periodic or constant pains, referred to the pelvic viscera, and dependent either upon inflammatory, congestive, or neurotic conditions, uterine or ovarian displacements, often yield in the happiest manner to galvanism—anode to painful points, cathode external—or to faradization according to Apostoli. This writer regards even acute perimetric inflammations as not contraindicating the employment of the faradic current. In the acute stages the bipolar vaginal electrode should be used; when the inflammation has somewhat subsided the intra-uterine current

Fig. 239.—Murray's Ovarian Electrode. should be brought into requisition. The measure of the strength of the faradic current used should be the sensation of the patient. The sittings may continue from five to twenty minutes, or until the patient expresses some sense of relief from pain. Sittings should be daily or twice a day.

Endometritis.—In this affection, likewise, Apostoli has made a distinct advance by his method of using strong electrolytic, or, as he terms them, chemical galvano-caustic currents. In cases attended by much haemorrhage or other discharge, he uses the positive pole in the uterus and the negative to the abdomen. In other cases the poles are reversed. This method is See *infra.* based upon the well-known fact, before referred to, that the positive pole of the galvanic current arrests haemorrhage; hence, Apostoli calls it the haemostatic pole.

As an intrauterine electrode he employs a sound insulated to near the point by means of a celluloid cannula, which is

Fig. 240.—Goblet's Intra-uterine Electrodes. pushed over the sound. The exposed portion of the sound must be of platinum or gold, in order to resist the action of the fluids when used as the positive pole. Dr. A. H. Goelet has recently described a uterine electrode made of steel, treated by a peculiar process, which is said to render it non-corrosive. This electrode with interchangeable tips is shown in Fig. 240. It can be used either as cathode or anode, and is much cheaper than a platinum or gold sound, and more durable than gold or aluminium.

The external electrode employed by Apostoli is a large, soft plate of clay, which is applied over the abdomen and con

Fig. 241.—Apostolus Abdominal Clay Electrode, With Contact-plate And Zinc Tray For Keeping The Clay Moist. nected as anode or cathode, accordingly as the negative or positive pole is in the uterine cavity. This electrode is made large and applied snugly to the surface of the abdomen, in order to thoroughly diffuse the current as it passes through the skin, and prevent any destructive effects at that point. The clay electrode of Apostoli (Fig. 241) is somewhat awkward to handle, and various modifications of it have been suggested or employed.

Fig. 242 shows Goelct's clay electrode, which is more cleanly and less inconvenient to handle. The clav is first worked to the consistence of putty, then rolled out into a flat cake and enveloped in a layer of absorbent cotton, covered with linen crash. A back of soft rubber is applied, by means of which it can be handled, and the patient's clothing kept dry. The metal contact-plate is pressed into the clay under the cotton. By means of a binding-post attached to this plate the electrode is connected with the connecting cords.

Another abdominal electrode for use in the Apostoli treatment is one devised by Dr. Franklin H. Martin, of Chicago, and

Fig. 243.—Martin's Abdominal Electrode. made by the Mcintosh Faradic and Battery Company (Fig. 243). It consists of a nickel-plated concave plate, covered with a membrane and having an insulated rim to prevent contact between the metal surface and the skin. When used, about a pint of warm water is poured into the receptacle formed by the concave plate and the membrane, through the nozzle shown in the figure. The membrane allows the transudation of sufficient liquid to keep it moist, and, as nothing but water is used, the apparatus is exceedingly cleanly. Dr. Martin claims that a very powerful current can be used with this electrode without producing any pain or destructive effects upon the skin.

The strength of current employed by Apostoli and other gynaecologists who have adopted his procedure is from 100 to 250 milliamperes. The duration of the sitting is from three to ten minutes. After the application there is often a sanguineous discharge from the uterus for several days, but there is rarely much febrile reaction if antiseptic precautions have been observed. The applications may be repeated once every week or ten days. The number of sittings required for the cure of the affection varies from three to thirty, according to the chronicity of the case.

Menorrhagia and Metrorrhagia.—These conditions or symptoms are frequently dependent upon endometritis, fibroid tumors, subinvolution, periuterine inflammations, or malignant growths of the uterus. In the first three the intra-uterine electrolytic method, above described, is usually beneficial. The positive pole arrests the haemorrhage. When due to periuterine inflammations, or merely to a relaxed condition of the uterine tissues, faradization is indicated. In some forms of malignant disease of the uterus electrolysis may be taken advantage of as a haemostatic, as well as for its trophic effects. *Inflammation of the Uterine and Periuterine Tissues and Uterine Appendages (Metritis, Peri-and Para-metritis, Salpingitis, Salpingo-ovaritis).*—Apostoli uses the faradic current in this class of inflammatory affections. No stage of the inflammation, even the most acute, contra-indicates the employment of the current. During the acute stage the bipolar vaginal electrode (Fig. 238) is used, being applied against the area of severest local pain.

After the acute symptoms have subsided the intra-uterine bipolar electrode (Fig. 237) is substituted. The sittings last from five to twenty minutes, and should not be terminated until the patient declares of her own volition that the pain is diminished. Strict antiseptic measures should be carried out before, during, and after the applications. The sittings may be repeated daily, or twice a day when the pain is severe.

After the pain has been for the most part relieved,—that is, when the case may be said to be in the chronic stage,—the galvanic current is substituted, using the positive pole in the uterus. The intra-uterine electrode of Apostoli, Fry, or Goelet may be used. Externally, the dispersion electrode for large currents (Apostoli's, Goelet's, or Martin's) may be applied. At first mild currents, 10 to 30 milliamperes, and sittings of two to *a Via.* 2-M.—Goblet's Uterine Puncture Needle. three minutes' duration twice a week should be employed. The strength of the applications and duration of the sittings may gradually be increased.

When the inflammatory symptoms have subsided entirely, and the exudation, serum, pus, or plastic material alone remains, the next step of the procedure arrives, namely, galvano-puncture. This is made from the vagina after an antiseptic irrigation, endeavoring to strike the tumor at its most depending part in order to secure free drainage. The platinum needle-electrode of Apostoli with a celluloid cannula as insulating guard, or a modification of the same by Dr. Goelet (Fig. 244), which is much cheaper, may be used. The insulating cover, B, is movable, and may be fixed at any position by the set-screw, C. In this way the depth to which the spear shall penetrate can be definitely fixed before the puncture is made. Goelet prefers to use a speculum to make the puncture, but Apostoli and other practitioners think this unnecessary. The puncture is made about a quarter of an inch in depth, and the posterior *cul-de-sac* is the point of election.

In his latest paper ipon this subject, Apostoli gives a careful review of his experience for the last seven years and full statement of his method of application. His conclusions are as follow:—

"1. Faradization, under the form of a current of tension, made by the long, thin wire, calms the nervous system, moderates its excitability, assuages or cures pain, but is often powerless to arrest an acute phlegmasia; its action is purely dynamic, and it acts, as opium acts, during early inflammatory stages, but is powerless to arrest the evolution of inflammatory processes. The current (faradic) of tension is the only one tolerable, and indicated in acute and subacute forms. A current of quantity is less efficacious and less tolerable, except in rare cases of chronic exudates, where, in acting upon the interstitial circulation, it aids re-absorption to a certain extent. The electrode should generally be the bipolar, to better localize the electric action, either in the vagina or in the uterus. All other things being equal, the uterine application is by far the most useful. The application should be in moderate doses without shock, and more gentle as the inflammation is more active. The *seances* should be daily at first, lasting from five to twenty minutes, and the dose progressively augmented as the patient can bear it.

"2. Galvanization, or," rather, intrauterine chemical caustique, is much more powerful than faradization, and will often be sufficient of itself in cases of ovaro-salpingitis. It is a most excellent way of changing in part or in whole the entire lining membrane of the uterus, and of setting up peripheric changes by derivation. The faradic current excites the nervous and muscular systems after the manner of a mechanical force, by interruptions and shocks. The galvanic current, however, is a physical and chemical force, at once caloric and trophic; and brings each of its factors into action separately or together, as desired. All binary compounds and those of greater complication will tend to decomposition, and this decomposition, called electrolysis, will be in proportion to the electric energy given out, and to the length of time of the application. This interstitial breaking up of the elements, which will be preceded by a different orientation in the polarization of the organic molecules, tends, on the one hand, to bring around the positive pole the acids and oxygen, while the bases and nitrogen go to the negative pole. Applied in a given region the galvanic current acts locally and generally; each pole has its undivided caustic action—the one acid, the other basic. The current is felt in the interpolar zone, engendering trophic changes, and tending to the resolution of certain pathological conditions.

The Treatment of Salpingo-Ovaritis by Electricity. *Journ. Am. Med. Asa'n,* July 27,1889.

"The doctor of to-day who has not kept apace with the advance of gynaecological science lauds to his utmost the curette, which first saw the light in France, but has long since fallen into desuetude in the land that originated it. Without wishing to discredit a surgical procedure of value in certain conditions, the superior advantages of the intrauterine galvanic current are beyond dispute.

"(a) It is simple and easy of application, requiring no assistant, and may be used by any one, no matter how little experience he has in gynaecology.

"(ft) Being but slightly painful, chloroform is not needed, this being only demanded in certain'cases of puncture.

"(c) It is valuable among working-women, as a short period of repose alone is necessary after the application, instead of hours and perhaps days in bed.

"(d) It can be gradually and gently applied by progressively increasing the strength, and is less brutal than the curette.

"(e) It is not contra-indicated in any acute case of inflammation, the sole caution being to use extra care, and to increase the strength only as the patient is able to bear it.

"(/) It is an agent which, instead of being blind, obeys in a precise and mathematical manner the hand applying it; that is to say, one can measure and administer it, and at the same time have an exact record of the amount of cauterization produced, to which three things conduce: the general intensity made use of, the density of the active electrode, and the duration of the application.

"(#) It is an active foree, which will produce an active result localizable at will, and which may be concentrated upon any part of the uterine lining-membrane desired.

"(h) It is absolutely harmless if proper antiseptic or aseptic precautions are made use of.

"(«') According to the intensity and duration its action can be varied, and also according to the active pole made use of; it may be made acid by using the positive pole and basic by using the negative pole.

"(j) Apart from the curetting action of the chemical galvanism, which one can easily sec, there is a more profound action, trophic and vital, and which is propagated along the whole organic circuit between the two poles. Thanks to this last consideration, above all in the treatment of salpingo-ovaritis, this chemical galvanism has a power far above surgical curetting, chiefly in reaching the uterine parenchyma and adnexa.

"(&) If surgical *rdcktge* often results in

frequent returns of the disease, causing anatomical and functional troubles which it hoped to combat, I can affirm that these results are much less frequent by the electrolytic treatment, which may require several *seances* to produce a lasting effect, but which good results, as I have had reason to observe in my clinic, last for many years after the cessation of all treatment.

"The operative technique is already sufficiently well explained in my various brochures upon the electric treatment of fibroma and endometritis. I shall content myself with giving you merely the salient features of the treatment of ovaro-salpingitis. The positive pole always causes less congestion than the negative, but the latter is more valuable to promote resolution. The positive pole should be used generally in the commencement, and, once having passed the first stage of toleration, the negative pole should be substituted. The dominant preoccupation which should make us cautious in treating salpingo-ovaritis, and which is sometimes difficult of recognition, is the fear of finding ourselves in the presence of a pyosalpinx, which a large dose of galvanism would aggravate; so, when in doubt, begin very gently with a mild current to test the susceptibility of the uterus and periuterine tissues, then increase with the patient's tolerance and according to clinical indications. One may begin with 20 to 40 milliampercs. If the intolerance is great, respect it and do not increase; if well tolerated, increase from 100 to 150 milliampercs. Here clinical diagnosis must be called in to differentiate between hysterical intolerance that need not be heeded and an inflammatory intolerance which must be respected. The sittings should not be too frequent. In the initial treatments they are frequently followed with a reaction more or less intense, which may last several days; generally we should wait until calm is re-established. Sometimes the *seances* may be given once or twice a week, sometimes only every fifteen days. The same reasons must guide the doctor as to the length of a *seance;* sometimes they should last three minutes, and sometimes five to eight minutes.

"3. I now come to the third division, the most efficacious of all, the penetration with the galvanic current of one of the vaginal *cul-de-sacs* at the nearest point of the inflamed region. I mean *vaginal galoano-puncture.* There are two clinical indications, the one of *choice,* the other of *necessity.* The indication of choice presents itself when one finds himself in presence of a salpingo-ovaritis which has not been sufficiently ameliorated by the intra-uteiine galvanism. It is necessary then to penetrate the mass in the point the nearest possible to the diseased spot, in order to lose nothing of electric force, which now should seriously concern itself with the suffering point. Theoretically the application, well made, should be most efficacious, and no doubt rests in my mind that such is the case, for the reply of all the patients who have submitted to this plan is that the punctures were much more painful but much more efficacious, because often one puncture gives more relief than many simple intra-uterine applications. The indication of *necessity* for galva no-puncture is when a fluctuating tumor impinges upon the vagina, and which should be drained antiseptically through the vagina.

"Already many years ago I gave the rules for the essentials of galvano-puncture. I will only now cite the chief points:—

"(a) Here, as in all electrical treatment, be it faradic or galvanic, one should precede everything with thorough antisepsis, preceding and following every operation with an antiseptic vaginal irrigation, either of sublimate, carbolic acid, creoline, or naphthol. Between the *seances* we shall do well to close the vaginal cavity with iodoform gauze (or sublimate or salol gauze), to insure perfect asepsis, as well as to prevent sexual congress, which should be suspended.

"*(b)* With the preceding electrical treatment it is not necessary to remain in bed. I exact from my patients only one or two hours of repose after galvano-caustique, without denying, however, that a longer period might be beneficial. Galvanopuncture, however, requires at least three days of rest in bed after each puncture.

"(c) The trocar carrying the current should be the smallest possible, but of sufficient resistance not to be easily broken. Steel is the best, because it penetrates easily.

"(f?) The chief point is the depth of the puncture. A slight puncture of *a half-centimetre,* as an average, suffices to make a door of entrance for the current in the region which it is to traverse. Deeper punctures do not suffice any better to attain such an end; on the contrary, as I have seen, they may be dangerous. I proscribe all punctures over one centimetre.

"(e) Where make the puncture"? Questions of choice and necessity here come up. The choice is to puncture as near as possible the diseased portion, but necessity forces us to avoid at all cost the anterior *cul-de-sac* on accoxint of the bladder. The lateral, and, above all, the posterior regions are the most favorable for the puncture. I make them oftenest in the posterior *cid-de-sac,* in the middle of the pouch of Douglas, directing the axis of the instrument toward the uterus in order to avoid the rectum.

"(/) This operation, much more painful than galvanocaustique, is often tolerated by certain women, but in others chloroform will be required.

"(/) *1 never use a speculum* in this operation, which can only be well and delicately carried out as follows: One fixes at first the exact length of the puncture, by turning the screw and advancing the steel point to the required length beyond the cellnloid; then, having fixed with the index finger the exact point to be punctured, and having made sure that there is no arterial pulsation, one slides the celluloid up to the point, which serves as the conductor for the trocar, which is then plunged in.

"(A) The number of punctures demanded is variable. Some cases of hydro and catarrhal salpingitis yield to one puncture, some require three or four, and tubercular tubes even more.

"Generally these cases require much longer periods of intermediate repose than cases of galvano-caustique, because at their commencement they are often followed by a severe reaction, which may last many days. The application should not be renewed until all the symptoms have disappeared.

"(i) As to intensity and choice of poles I repeat what I said just now when speaking of intra-uterine galvanization. The intensity will vary from 20 to 50 milliamperes. To go beyond this is to go beyond the point of tolerance, and chloroform should be used. To create a temporary vaginal fistula 100 to 250 milliamperes will be required.

"(j) The puncture should generally be positive at first, because it is more tolerable and less exciting than the negative. This latter is employed when a more powerful action is demanded. Especially in presence of a fluctuating tumor pointing into the vagina, in which a fistulous tract is to be made and vaginal drainage established, is the negative pole demanded.

"*(k)* Should febrile excitement arise all treatment is to be suspended. One may think himself in the presence of pyosalpinx if it points into the vagina, and a puncture is not contraindicated; but if it is high up, not accessible, and far from the vaginal *cul-de-sac,* a deep puncture, which might cause an evacuation into the cavity of the peritoneum of the sac, is to be avoided. It is here that surgery must step in to carry out its legitimate functions.

"My clinical experience, which is now seven years old, has given me many cases of salpingo-ovaritis, which I hope later on to tabulate. I shall content myself now with some results of my treatment. Every salpingo-ovaritis will generally be suitable for appropriate electrical treatment, and this should be the conservative method of choice; it is sovereign in catarrhal salpingitis, only calmative in tubercular salpingo-ovaritis, and in certain pus-tubes may be of great service. Whatever electric treatment is made use of, it should be continued until the patient pronounces herself cured of her symptoms, and until an examination has satisfied us that the anatomical change is considerable. Surgical interference should never be resorted to until after all electrical resources have been exhausted. Castration, which morally and physically mutilates a woman after an incurable fashion, and only cures radically in a fourth or fifth part of the cases, should be only an operation of necessity, never of choice, and should be regarded as a last resort. Electrical conservative therapeusis, harmless, easily applied by any one, and which does not pretend to cure every case of salpingoovaritis, finds its greatest triumph in rendering a *subsequent conception* possible, as I have seen in several of my patients." *Uterine Displacements.*—Reference has already been made to Apostoli's treatment of flexion by means of faradization, and the application of the constant current for the same purpose. Other forms of displacement, especially if due to relaxation of the muscular structures of the vagina and uterine ligaments, are also susceptible to electrical treatment. Faradization would seem to be most rationally indicated, as it not only improves the contractility of the muscular elements in the ligaments, but also relieves congestion of the uterus and other pelvic organs and tissues. Lumbo-abdominal, utero-spinal, or utero-abdominal currents may be tried. In using the galvanic current care must be taken to avoid the cauterizing action of the pelvic electrode.

Uterine Tumors.—Eighteen years ago Drs. Ephraim Cutter and Gilman Kimball operated upon a case of fibroid tumor of the uterus by passing a galvanic current through portions of the morbid growth, using insulated needles as electrodes. The question of priority in suggesting and performing the operation does not seem to have been definitely settled between these two gentlemen. At the Washington International Medical Congress of 1887 both claimed the honor. Dr. Cutter has, since that time, operated in a large number of cases, and, in 1887, reported fifty cases with the following results: 25 arrests; 7 non-arrests; 3 relieved; 11 cured; 4 deaths. These results are fairly good. While the number of cures is small, and the deaths comparatively large (8 per cent.), the showing is much more satisfactory than either medical treatment or hysterectomy. In 1884 Dr. Apostoli published the results of a new method of electrical treatment of uterine fibroids. The method has. been extensively discussed in the journals the past five years, and has given rise to much acrimonious debate.

In Great Britain, Sir Spencer Wells, Thomas and Skene Keith, Dr. W. S. Playfair, W. E. Steavenson, and many others have adopted Apostolus method and claim for it advantages over any other now in use for treating this class of morbid growths. In America the prominent adherents among gynaecologists are I.. Carlct: T)u traitem. Electr. dea tumeurs flbreuses do l'ute'rus d'aprfcs, la lue'thodc du Dr. Apo9toli. Paris, 18S4.

as yet few, but there are signs of yielding, and it will probably not be very long before the electrical treatment of fibroids becomes as popular in this country as it is in England.

The method is essentially the same as that for treating chronic perimetric inflammations as above described. The procedures consist of the use of the positive electrode in the cavity of the uterus in cases where haemorrhage is a marked symptom (positive chemical galvanocauterization); the negative electrode intra-utcrine to promote absorption (negative chemical galvanocauterization), and negative puncture of the tumor through the cervix or vagina (negative galvano-puncture). The currents used are strong (from 50 to 250 milliamperes) and the sittings from two to five minutes in duration. The intra-uterine applications may be repeated once or twice a week. The external electrode used is the clay diffusion electrode for the abdomen.

The results claimed for the treatment are:— 1. Arrest of hemorrhage.
2. Cessation of pain. 3. Diminution in size of the tumor.

Complete disappearance of the tumor is rare, although it has sometimes occurred alter puncture.

When the cervix is too tortuous to get the sound into the uterus, or is obliterated by the growth, a new canal is made by means of galvano-puncture. This canal is said to remain patulous, and all intra-uterine applications are made through it.

In July, 1887, Apostoli reported two hundred and seventyeight cases treated by this method, making upward of four thousand applications, an average of about fifteen applications in each case. Benefit is claimed in about 95 *per cent,* of the cases. The cases are "symptomatieally cured," *i. e.,* the symptoms for which the patients sought relief have been alleviated or entirely removed, although the tumor had not disappeared. By some it is asserted that this relief is only temporary, but even then it is better than doing nothing or, perhaps, as is the case with some gynaecologists with surgical tendencies, doing too much.

Among the latest contributions in favor of the electrolytic treatment of fibroid tumors is a paper by Thomas Keith, who, although his success in treating these growths with the knife stands unparalleled, has become the strongest advocate of Apostolus treatment. He closes his paper with the following strong statement:—

"The only treatment not surgical worth speaking about that I have seen do any good, and which, at the same time, is one free from danger to life if the treatment be undertaken by one who has respect jbr a strong electrical current, is that brought before us by Dr. Apostoli. If any one should have held on firmly to hysterectomy it is myself, for my results after it are better than any other. I have, however, thrown over all surgical operations for this new treatment, and the longer I follow it the more am I satisfied

"To the surgeon, no doubt, hysterectomy is the good and simple plan. He may have his bad quarter of an hour at the operation, but then he has practically done with the case, and he gets his result quickly, sometimes more quickly than he cares for. If the patient recover there is pleasure all around; if things go badly and the patient die, he bewails his bad luck, as it is called,.... waits a little, and then, though rather unwillingly, does another. He resents any other treatment than that by the knife. He especially resents Apostoli's treatment of fibroids by electricity, for the result is long in coming; it is a slow treatment, requiring great patience, great tenderness of manipulation, and much thinking But with patience the result is certain There is no mutilation, a thing abhorrent to most women It puts a woman with a fibrous tumor, who suffers much, into the. position of a woman with a fibrous tumor who does not suffer or may be even unaware of its presence. It does not bring about the disappearance of the tumor, or it does so very rarely, but the size is lessened more or less—one-half, one-third, two-thirds

Tension is taken off everywhere, all around, and bladder irritability from pressure, a common cause of distress, is relieved. In a word, the woman is made well; her whole life is changed. All this can be done without danger to life, and if there be pain during the time the current passes the fault is in the operator. What more does a reasonable woman who has suffered much desire or need?

"What have those to offer in place of all this who have so bitterly opposed this treatment; who with unlimited material stand aside and will not take the trouble to investigate the matter for themselves, but wait till some one else does it for them; who make only an outcry if by chance they hear of any accident during the progress of the treatment of any case, and who go frantic over the rumor of a death, or, worse still, who proclaim they know of deaths that never happen These men have absolutely nothing whatever to offer in the bad cases, and only *hysterectomy in such tumors that will come out more or less easily,* so as to be treated by the extra-peritoneal method of operating. I have seen not a few cases of bad bleeding fibroids since I came to London; almost every one had consulted one or other surgical authority on the subject of operation. These were invariably told that nothing would do them any good but the removal of the tumor; but in their special case the local difficulties were too great, or they had let their strength go down too far for such an operation. The very feeble and bad cases, with masses of tumor blocking the pelvis, with absence of cervix, and opened-out broad ligaments, would seem to be let alone. Hysterectomy, then, at best, would appear to be a most doubtful remedy for a certain number of cases, and these not of the worst sort. On the other hand, the worse the case, the more feeble the patient, the greater the loss of blood, the more marked is the result of electrical treatment. Given a woman with a large bleeding fibroid, blanched almost to death from years of haemorrhage, and see her some months after this treatment is completed, you would scarcely recognize her,—the improvement is so great

"The old spirit that at one time would have no abdominal surgery still, unfortunately, lingers among us. Electricity in any form, when applied to the cure of disease, is set down as pure quackery by many medical men, simply because they know nothing about it, and won't take the trouble to learn for themselves what to many is rather a hard study...

"What I now plead for is that, for a time, all bloody operations for the treatment of uterine fibroids should cease, and that Dr. Apostoli's treatment, as practiced by him, should have a fair trial. Those who have hitherto most resisted the introduction of electricity are the surgeons who are the best competent to carry it out. They are accustomed to manipulate in the pelvis, and they will not make mistakes in the diagnosis, or make them as seldom as it is possible to do. Hysterectomy, remember, which is performed every day for a complaint that rarely of itself shortens life, kills every fourth or fifth woman who is subjected to it. This mortality must cease; it is not a question of surgery,—it is a question of humanity. Every time that any disease can be cured without resorting to a bloody operation, such as hysterectomy, progress is made in our art, and there is a gain to humanity, while surgery is the better for being purged of a deadly operation. It may seem strange to some that after the results I got in hysterectomy—results that almost made it justifiable—I should now begin to throw stones at the operation instead of trying still further to improve upon it; and but for Dr. Apostoli I would now be doing so. I would give something to have back again those sixty-four women that I did hysterectomy for, that I might have a trial of Dr. Apostoli's treatment upon them; and I would give something never to have had the wear and tear of flesh and spirit that these operations cost me, for in scarcely one of them was the operation simple."

Testimony like this is certainly valuable in favor of an operation so simple and so little fraught with danger to life. Apostoli in two hundred and seventy-eight cases lost two, and Keith in a large number but one.

Dr. Franklin H. Martin, of Chicago, has described what he claims to be a new method of electrical treatment of uterine fibroids, but which appears to be merely a trivial modification of Apostoli's method. The modifications of some of the instruments used seem to be desirable improvements, but no distinct advance is discernible in the procedure.

Fig. 245.—Carbon-disk Electrode For Vagina.

Malignant tumors of the uterus have not been subjected to electrolysis, although the results obtained with more superficial growths of the kind should encourage a trial of the method in carcinoma and sarcoma. Epithelioma of the os and cervix could be readily treated by electrolysis if a proper electrode were constructed for the purpose. The carbon-disk electrode of Dr. Goelet (Fig. 245) would seem particularly appropriate for some cases of epitheliomatous ulceration of the os uteri.

Amputation of the cervix for epithelioma and hypertrophy is often performed with galvano-cautery. The apparatus re

Fig. 216.—Large Screw-cautery Handle. quired, in addition to a proper cautery battery and wire snare, is a large screw electrode to slowly tighten the wire as it is being heated (Fig. 246).

Ovarian Tumors.—While the electrolytic treatment of uterine fibroids may be considered to be fairly on trial, that of ovarian cysts has not been able to obtain recognition from the profession. Dr. Semeleder, of Mexico, who has practiced the method for a number of years, has recently published the results of his experience, which docs not appear to be so unfavorable as it has been made to appear by Dr. Munde, in a contribution to the "Transactions of the American Gynaecological Society," for 1877. Dr. Munde's method of interpreting statistics has certainly the merit of originality, even though it lacks some of the elements of fairness, when he says in a later article: "I collected fifty-one cases, of which only twenty-eight might credibly be considered cured; nine died, and fourteen were utter failures. The ratio of mortality and failure was 45 *per cent.,* or double the mortality from ovariotomy, even in the hands of our less successful operators of to-day." The absolute mortality was 20 percent. Dr. Semeleder f reports his personal experience with electrolysis as follows: Of forty cases of ovarian cysts there were twenty-seven cured; three improved; one temporarily improved; in two there was no change; two were still under treatment, and five died. This gives an absolute mortality of 12.5 per cent. In 1887, Dr. Munde reports his own experience % with ovariotomy during the year as twenty-two operations with five deaths, a mortality of 22.7 per cent. Is Dr. Munde to be numbered among " our less successful operators *V* Transactions Ninth International Congress, vol. ii, p. 669-684.

Probably the best method of electrolysis of ovarian tumors would be, where possible, negative galvano-puncture from the vagina, with a large diffusion positive electrode on the abdomen. With proper antiseptic precautions the abdominal puncture would probably not be very dangerous. The method demands further study on the part of those who are in position and willing to give it the requisite attention.

Extra-uterine Pregnancy.—One of the most beneficent applications of electricity is in the destruction of foetal life in extra-uterine pregnancy. It is admitted by most obstetricians that if the diagnosis can be certainly made before the death of the foetus the electrical treatment is the most appropriate procedure. Until recently the possibility of making such a diagnosis has been generally accepted, but some surgeons who oppose the use of electricity now state that the diagnosis of ectopic pregnancy cannot be made before the life of the foetus is extinct, or the cyst in which it is contained has been ruptured. It is also argued that the placenta continues growing after the foetus dies, and hence the danger of internal haemorrhage still continues. am. Journ. of Obstetrics, December, 1885. t Wiener Klinik, Octo)er, 1888.

J Ooodell in Sajous' "Annual," for 1888, vol. iv, p. 106.

Unfortunately for these theoretical objections, (foetal) antemortem diagnosis of ectopic pregnancy has been made in a sufficient number of instances to establish its possibility, and the demonstration of the (foetal) post-mortem growth of the placenta has not yet been furnished.

In a considerable number of cases on record in the obstetrical literature success has followed the use of electricity in this grave condition. Among American authorities may be quoted Urs. T. Gaillard Thomas, W. T. Lusk, R. P. Harris, A. D. Rockwell, and others who have either had personal experience or approve the method. The faradic current is usually employed, one electrode being applied over the tumor externally and the other against the most prominent part of the swelling in the vagina. Daily sittings of ten minutes each, for two to three weeks, gradually increasing the strength of the current to the limit of endurance and then diminishing it to zero at each sitting, will usually destroy the foetal vitality if employed before the third month. In one of Lusk's cases the foetal vitality was evidently destroyed after six applications; in another, after ten; in a case reported by Dr. McBurney two applications, and in one by Dr. Billington four, sufficed to arrest the vitality of the foetus. In none of these cases were there any dangerous aftereffects, either from the applications or from the foetal structures and placenta which were allowed to remain in the cyst.

Some obstetricians prefer the galvanic current, and, *a priori*, it would seem to be the most appropriate, as the electrolytic effects would promote absorption of the contents of the sac. Dr. Rockwell uses an interrupted galvanic current, sending a succession of shocks through the sac. He uses a current strength of 10 to 30 milliamperes. In one case a single application was sufficient to arrest the embryonic life. In one case of advanced tubal pregnancy Dr. Thomas opened the sac from the vagina by means of the galvano-cautery.

Urethral Caruncle and Other Growths of the External Genitals.—Electrolysis or galvano-cautery under cocaine may be employed for the destruction of these new formations. It is probable that the tendency of the caruncular growths to return after extirpation with the knife would not attend their electrolytic destruction. *Atresia or Stenosis of the Vagina.*—Just as stricture of the urethra, rectum, and other mucous canals is amenable to electrolytic treatment, so in cases where the vagina is narrowed from cicatricial contraction, the same procedure may be expected to give relief. It would seem that in the preparatory treatment of vesico-vaginal fistula electrolysis is rationally indicated, not for the cure of fistula, but for the removal of the cicatricial and other obstructive conditions which so often interfere with the success of the recognized surgical procedures in these cases.
ELECTRICITY IN OBSTETRICS.

Abortion.—At first thought it appears contradictory-o use electricity for the prevention of abortion, but when it is considered that electricity, especially the faradic current, reduces local nervous irritability, it will be seen that a prime indication in this condition is fulfilled by this agent. Experienced obstetricians know that one of the best means to quiet an irritable uterus in threatened abortion is ergot in small doses. Electricity in mild currents produces similar "sedative" effects, and is hence rationally indicated in cases where abortion is threatened, but where the separation of the membranes is not yet extensive.

Dr. W. T. Baird, of Texas, takes a similar view of the effect of mild currents in this condition. He reports three cases "who were threatened with abortion, and who were having haemorrhage when the treatment was commenced; and in these three latter (he continues) the treatment was instituted to arrest the haemorrhage and prevent the expulsion of the ovum. The results justified my expectations in each case, as the haemorrhage was promptly arrested, and the patients all went over to full term." In these cases an insulated vaginal electrode was introduced into the vagina and pressed against the os, while a soft-sponge electrode was applied over the hypogastrium or the lumbosacral region for ten minutes. The faradic current was used.

To arrest haemorrhage from a relaxed uterus, after abortion, the same current may be employed either with the electrodes similarly applied or with a double uterine electrode (Fig. 247),

Fig. 247.—Double Uterine Electrode. by means of which the current can be definitely localized in the uterus, and produce more forcible contraction. The same instrument is exceedingly useful in post-partum haemorrhage. In haemorrhage after abortion, where there are retained membranes, the use of a negative galvanic pole in the uterus and a current of 50 to 60 milliamperes for five to ten minutes gives good results.

Puerperal Haemorrhage.—Haemorrhage before, during, or after labor at term is always an alarming sign. When it occurs before labor as an indication of placenta praevia, the induction of premature labor is demanded. When the bleeding comes on during or after labor there is no agent that can be relied upon with so much satisfaction as electricity. The faradic current, as strong as can be borne, should be used to produce strong, equable contractions of the muscular tissue, and thus arrest the bleeding. The current can be sent from back to abdomen, or from uterus to abdomen, or through the uterus alone, by means of the double uterine electrode. Am. Journ. of Obstetrics, April, 1885, p. 3U. *Premature Delivery.*—When premature delivery is indicated, one of the promptest methods to produce it is by means of electricity. Either the galvanic or faradic current may be employed, preference being generally given to the latter. Lumboabdominal currents, as strong as the patient can bear, are used. Under its influence the os begins to dilate and contractions begin in the organ which soon expel its contents. *Parturition.*—In the process of labor the administration of chloroform is a favorite method of allaying the pains, calming the nervousness, and securing personal quiet. Dr. Baird claims that a mild faradic current will produce a similar effect, relieving promptly all so-called "reflex pains," without diminishing the contractile or expulsive pains. His method is to apply a large electrode to the sacrum, and with a wristlet electrode (Fig. 248) attached to the operator's arm pass the hand over the abdomen during the pains. In this way the strength of the current can be readily regulated, the application is diffused over the abdomen, and a species of massage with the electric hand can be combined with the electricity. In place of the hand a large sponge may be used as the abdominal electrode.

Dr. Baird lays down the following indications for the use of electricity in obstetrics:—

"1. To modify the pains of labor.

12. To favor a more rapid dilatation of the os.

u

"3. To promote more vigorous uterine contractions.

"4. To add tone and strength to all the muscles engaged, and increase their power of doing work.

"5. To abridge the time occupied by the labor.

"6. To prevent shock, exhaustion, and post-partum haemorrhage.

"7. To insure contraction of the uterus in cases of instrumental delivery.

"8. To act as an auxiliary in the induction of premature labor.

"9. To arrest haemorrhage and accelerate labor in cases of placenta praevia.

"10. To prevent an undue expenditure of nervous force in all cases of debility from whatever cause, thus leaving the patient in a condition to secure a speedy and favorable convalescence."

Apostoli and Tripier use faradization after labor to promote involution of the uterus. The regular contraction thus produced acts in a measure as preventive of septic absorption by keeping the uterine cavity empty. The sittings may be repeated daily for one or two weeks, or longer if deemed necessary. The lumbo-abdominal method is generally sufficient to maintain good contraction of the womb.

DISEASES OF THE MALE GENITO-URINARY ORGANS.

Among the derangements of the male genito-urinary apparatus in which electricity may be used with good promise of success are various paretic conditions of the bladder and penis, irritability of the bladder and urethra, functional impotence, and certain consequences of inflammation in the urethral canal or contiguous tissues and organs. The galvanic and faradic currents and static electricity may be employed locally. In certain cases the effects of electricity upon the cerebro-spinal nervous system

Am. Jour. Obstetrics, July, 1885.

and upon the general nutrition of the organism may also be called to aid. *Irritability of the Urethra.*—In cases where there is an itching or tingling sensation in the urethra, which frequently deepens into positive pain during urination or seminal discharge, the galvanic current, with the negative electrode in the urethra and the positive upon the pubis or thigh, generally gives prompt relief. Currents of two to five milliamperes are sufficient, with sittings of five minutes' duration, once or twice a week. Faradization may be employed in the same manner. *Chronic Inflammation and Stricture of the Urethra.* — In chronic urethritis following gonorrhoea there is often a localized area of tenderness in the deep urethra, accompanied by a slight discharge. When a catheter or sound is passed it gives exquisite pain as it passes over the tender area referred to, and upon withdrawal of the instrument more or less bleeding follows— sometimes a few drops only of blood, at others quite a smart haemorrhage. There is good reason to believe that this painful area is in a granular condition, and the bleeding and reflex spasmodic contraction following attempts to pass a sound over it often lead the physician to the opinion that he has to deal with a stricture. Careful examination with a urethrameter or bulbous sound will demonstrate the absence of any organic co-arctation of the urethral calibre. In these cases no remedy will yield so prompt and satisfactory results as the galvanic current applied as directed for irritability of the urethra. An insulated sound somewhat smaller than the normal urethral calibre should first be used. This is attached as negative electrode and passed down the urethra until it strikes the painful point. The anode—ordinary contact electrode—is then applied to the thigh and the current gradually turned on until four or five milliamperes are passing. Very slight pressure in the appropriate direction is then made upon the sound, and in a few minutes it will be found to slip through the formerly contracted and painful portion of the canal and may be made to enter the bladder. The sound should then be slowly retracted without breaking the circuit until the painful area has been passed, when the circuit may be opened and the urethral electrode withdrawn. There will usually be a little bleeding and some pain, with a strong desire to urinate, which should be gratified. The penis, scrotum, and perinaeum should be bathed in hot water for a few minutes at a time four or five times after the operation. The sittings may be repeated once or twice a week, and should not exceed five minutes each. It needs no urging to use only the gentlest manipulation in introducing any kind of instrument into the urethra. After the first sitting the pain and bleeding become less until after three or four sittings they disappear entirely. Four to six weeks' treatment is usually sufficient for the cure of this affection. In urethral stricture the same method of treatment is pursued.

Fig. 249.—Insulated Uketural Sound.

The normal calibre of the urethra, the size and location of the stricture are first determined, and then an insulated sound (Fig. 249), connected as cathode, a little larger than the stricture, is passed down to the strictured portion of the canal.

The circuit is then closed, with the anode on the thigh, and the current gradually turned on with the rheostat or current selector. A strength of 4 to 8 milliamperes may be used. If the stricture is an infiltrated and not a cicatricial one, it will usually yield to very slight pressure in a few minutes. The sound should then be drawn backward slowly through the strictured portion of the canal, and then the circuit opened. No attempts should be made to pass a second larger instrument at the same sitting. Even if the sound used is too large, and will not pass the stricture within five minutes, it is better not to irritate the urethra by persistent trials with the same or a smaller electrode. The patient should be sent away with directions to bathe the penis and perinieum in hot water. Another attempt may be made in three or four days. If the sound has been properly chosen, and is appropriately handled, there will usually be little difficulty in passing the constricted area.

The number of sittings required to cure a strictured urethra by electrolysis depends upon so many modifying circumstances that no safe prediction can be made. In careful hands the number of sittings required will be from ten to twelve.

This method is the one usually practiced, and owes much of its popularity to the advocacy of Dr. Robert Newman, of New York, who has had very extensive practice with it. It fulfills all the indications presented by a stricture due to an infiltrated area of submucous connective tissue—the type of an inflammatory stricture. In strictures due to cicatricial tissue or to linear co-arctation, as sometimes found near the meatus, the method advocated by Dr. J. A. Fort seems better adapted. In this method the active portion of the electrode consists in a linear exposure of metal at or near the point of the sound. By the use of this instrument a narrow furrow can be ploughed through the constricted portion of the canal, and afterward dilatation, either with or without electricity, practiced. Dr. Fort also uses this method for all ordinary strictures, and reports satisfactory results with it.

It must be well understood that this operation is not in the nature of a cauterization; it is electrolysis pure and simple. There is no elevation of temperature in the electrode, and no charring of tissue. The pathological tissue is slowly dissolved by the electrolytic action of the current, which probably also stimulates the absorption of infiltrated products..

It is quite probable that some surgeons have failed with either of these methods, and cases doubtless occur in which urethrotomy is a quicker, safer, easier, and more effectual method of cure; but success with one method of treatment, and failure with another, does not give an operator the right to deny any merit to the latter, or to discredit the testimony of those whose experience has been different.

Galvano-cautery has also been practiced in some cases of urethral stricture, but the occasions on which it can be preferred to electrolysis must be very rare. In cicatricial strictures near the meatus it may be employed with success.

Paresis and Paralysis of the Bladder.—Paralytic conditions of the bladder may manifest themselves either by retention or incontinence of urine. They may also be due to cerebral, spinal, or peripheral nerve-lesions. In the former case galvanization of the brain and spinal cord is indicated. In most cases, indeed, galvanization of the lumbar cord is beneficial in addition to the local symptomatic treatment. The latter may consist in percutaneous, lumbo-abdominal, or lumbo-perineal galvanization, faradization, or the combined currents. Perhaps a better method is to introduce an insulated urethral electrode into the bladder, and pass a faradic current, with the external electrode against the perinaeum, the lumbar spine, or over the pubis. In this case the bladder should be filled with a weak saline (borax) solution, or be allowed to fill with urine, in order that the current may become well diffused. When there is paralysis of the neck of the bladder the current should be localized by holding the internal electrode in the vesical neck, and pressing the external electrode against the perinaeum, or introducing it into the rectum. The galvanic current may also be used as an intra-vesical current, introducing the cathode into the bladder, and applying the anode externally, either over the spine, perinaeum, or pubis. *Nocturnal Incontinence of Urine.* — This condition yields very readily to electricity. The faradic current is usually employed, although galvanism, likewise, gives good results. One insulated electrode is introduced a short distance into the urethra, and may be pushed up to the neck of the bladder; the other is applied over the pubis or spine. Percutaneous currents from the spine to the pubis are sometimes effective. Improvement usually follows after the first sitting. Galvanization of the spine is a useful adjunct to the local electrization. *Spermatorrhoea, Involuntary Seminal Emissions, and Functional Impotence.*—In all of these conditions intra-urethral galvanization and faradization are of benefit. In emissions the internal electrode should be placed against the mouths of the seminal ducts, and the external to the perinaeum. Mild galvanic currents (2 to 4 milliamperes), with cathode in the urethra, will often arrest the discharges by relieving the irritability of the urethra. Faradization may be used in the same way, and in addition transverse faradization of the testicles and spinal galvanization are of benefit. In impotence (deficient erectile power) spinal galvanization and galvano-faradization from the lumbar spine to the penis and scrotum give the best promise of success. The dry faradic brush to the penis, scrotum, and inner sides of the thighs is also at times an efficient method of producing erections. Electric baths are occasionally useful. *Hypertrophy of the Prostate.*—Faradization by means of an insulated sound in the urethra and another in the rectum has been used with success by Tripier. When the prostatic portion of the urethra will not admit an instrument Tripier uses a double bulbous rectal electrode, which is pressed forward against the prostate so as to apply itself to either side of the latter and the current passed through the enlarged organ from side to side. Galvanism can be employed in a similar manner. Cheron and Moreau-Wolf claim good success with the cathode pressed well against the prostate from the rectum and the anode to the perinaeum. Fort's linear electrolytic method would doubtless gradually plough a furrow through the enlarged middle lobe if a sufficiently strong current, say 5 to 10 milliamperes, were used. Newman has devised a cautery electrode (Fig. 250) which he uses for the purpose of destroying the obstruction in the canal. The sound with the platinum-wire burner at e is passed down to the obstruction, and then by means of the key. b, the circuit is closed and the wire heated to a red heat. A cautery battery is used. The burning must be done very quickly in order not to destroy deeply and leave a slough. The method is said to be painless, and sittings may be repeated once a week. It seems that in addition to the destruction of tissue this method causes certain modifications of nutrition, followed by absorption of part of the hypertrophied growth.

Very recently a new procedure for reducing the size of an hypertrophied prostate by electrolysis has been proposed by Dr. Casper, of Berlin, who reports four cases, of which two were cured. He employs a needle-electrode as cathode, which is plunged into the prostate from the rectum. The needle is insulated to near its point. The anode is applied over the pelvis. A current of from 10 to 25 milliamperes is used. The sittings may be repeated every five or six days. The method seems worthy of further trial. It is said not to be painful unless a greater current strength than 15 milliamperes is used.

Chronic Orchitis.—The swollen testicle should be subjected to transverse percutaneous galvanization. Lewandowski has succeeded with the electrodes thus placed, and frequently reversing the current. Galvanization of the spermatic cord is practiced in addition. *Atrophy of the Testicle.*—Faradization of the testicle and spermatic cord may prove successful. *Varicocele.*—In this affection electrolysis with the anode in the vein to produce coagulation seems rationally indicated. The possibility of detachment of the clot and consequent pulmonary embolism must, however, be borne in mind. *Hydrocele.*—Both the faradic and galvanic currents may cause absorption of the effusion in hydrocele. The faradic current is employed percutaneously. The galvanic current may be applied in the same way, or by puncturing the sac with the cathode and using a pretty strong current (30 to 50 milliamperes) to produce electrolysis.

DISEASES OF THE GLANDS.

In the treatment of glandular enlargements by electricity the galvanic current is usually employed, the current being passed through the uninjured skin (percutaneous method) or one or both poles armed with insulated needles may be plunged into the growth (galvano-puncture, electrolysis).

Cataphoric transmission of absorbent medicines (iodine) has been employed with asserted success, in some cases. Faradic currents passed through the glands, or by means of the faradic brush, to stimulate absorption by reflex action upon the absorbents, have also been successfully used.

Enlarged Lymphatic Glands.—Excellent results have been obtained in enlarged lymphatic glands by the use of the galvanic current, either percutaneously or by means of negative galvanopuncture. When the enlargement is due to specific infective processes, or suppuration has taken place, the procedure is likely to fail. Broken-down glands may, however, readily be opened by means of negative galvano-puncture when the patient objects

Fig. 351.—Wire Cautery Point. to incision. Galvano-cautery is a favorite method of opening glands. It is thoroughly aseptic, and the interior of the cavity may be readily cauterized by the cautery point. In some cases, such as enlarged tonsils, both the galvano-cautery and electrolysis have decided advantages over any other mode of treatment. If the cautery is used the wire point (Fig. 251) may be employed, a number of punctures being made with it into the substance of the gland. The sittings may be repeated weekly or bi-weekly. The hypertrophied gland-substance is partly destroyed and partly condensed by the small contractile cicatrices produced. In electrolytic puncture with the negative needle we have an equally effective method, but much more tedious.

The proper strength of the current in electrolysis of glands is from 5 to 20 milliamperes. Sittings should last from five to ten minutes and may be repeated once or twice a week. The needles should always be kept thoroughly aseptic in order to avoid inducing suppuration. M. Meyer employs strong, frequently-interrupted faradic currents in enlarged lymphatic glands, and reports good results therefrom.

Goitre.—In a moderate proportion of cases the percutaneous method of employing galvanism is successful. Chvostek, Bruns, and Lewandowski cured about 15 per cent, of their cases. Rapid diminution of the tumor is often observed, but unless the treatment is continued for some time the growth is liable to again enlarge. The method is to place large, moist electrodes on each side of the tumor, and pass a current of 10 to 20 milliamperes. The electrodes should be frequently moved to avoid destroying the skin by electrolytic action. Another method is to apply one electrode over the tumor and the other in the auriculo-maxillary angle. The relative position of the poles seems to have little influence, but most practitioners apply the cathode over the growth.

Negative galvano-puncture with one or more insulated needles and' a current of 5 to 10 milliamperes, weekly or semi-weekly sittings, may also be employed. By this method improvement is almost certain to follow, although, as with other methods, failures must be expected.

The treatment by electrolysis is neither painful nor dangerous.

Multiple punctures with the galvano-cautery wire may also be expected to give good»results. The destruction of skin-tissue will, however, cause numerous small scars, which can be avoided in electrolysis by using insulated needles.

Agalactia.—Deficient action of the mammary gland is a disorder comparatively frequent. It often yields promptly to faradic stimulation. Large, moist electrodes are applied directly to the breast. Static electricity has been used successfully for the same purpose. *Indurations of the Mammary Gland.*— The indurations following chronic inflammation and abscess of the mammary gland will often undergo rapid absorption under the influence of galvanism. Large, moist electrodes are applied in a manner that the current will pass through the gland. In acute inflammation of the gland, before the formation of pus, the pain and tension can be relieved by the faradic current. *Tumors.*—Dr. A. C. Garratt has reported one hundred and fifty-seven cures out of one hundred and eighty-six tumors of the breast treated with the galvanic current. The tumors (or indurations) are inclosed between two sponge electrodes (two by three inches area) and a current varying in strength from 5 to 50 milliamperes used.

Epitheliomata of the breast have been extirpated by electrolysis, but the method is tedious and generally unsatisfactory. It is possible that in the early period of the growth the persistent use of the percutaneous galvanic current will prove successful.

Very recently, Dr. J. Inglis Parsonsf reported four cases of cancer in which the progress of the disease was arrested by strong currents of electricity passed through the growth. Currents varying from 10 to 600 milliamperes, with an electro-motive force of 105 volts, were used, the tumor being transfixed with fine insulated needles. The patients were anaesthetized during the operation. A nodular mass of fibrous tissue remains. The Trans. Ninth Intern. Med. Congress, vol. it t Brit. Med. Journ.,

April 27, 1889.
observations of Dr. Parsons are an encouragement to further experiment in this direction. There is reason to believe that the limitations of electrical treatment of malignant tumors have not yet been reached.

DISEASES OF THE SKIN.

In skin diseases of neurotic origin the use of electricity is rationally indicated, and is often effectual. In inflammatory affections the galvanic current may likewise be often used with good results. Certain subjective symptoms, as pain, itching, hyperesthesia, etc., are frequently promptly relieved by the faradic or galvanic current. General electrization by means of electric baths and static electricity (insulation and breeze) are indicated in certain general neuroses with cutaneous manifestations.

Angioneuroses.—(Edema, urticaria, and neurotic bullous eruptions are successfully aborted by means of the galvanic current, the anode being applied to the spine and the cathode to the seat of the outbreak. The itching of urticaria, eczema, lichen, and prurigo may frequently be promptly, though not permanently, relieved by swelling faradic currents.

Chilblains often yield to galvanization and faradization. In the early stages of local asphyxia (Raynaud's disease) the angiospasm may be arrested by a strong faradic current, and the normal circulation re-established. In more advanced cases, when trophic changes of the skin have begun, galvanism, with the cathode to the affected area, may be useful, and in the absence of any other trustworthy remedy should be faithfully tried.

In most cases of neurotic skin diseases, spinal, central, and subaural galvanization should be employed in addition to the local applications of the current.

Eczema. — Beard and Rockwell recommend very highly central galvanization in this disease. Local faradization and galvanization (anode to eruption) also give good results, promptly relieving the itching and reducing hyperemia. In chronic cases with much infiltration the galvanic current, using the cathode to the seat of eruption, is rationally indicated. *Psoriasis and Lichen Planus.*—Looking upon these diseases as in a measure neurotic in origin, spinal and central galvanization should give relief. The reported successes with the remedy are, however, very few in number, and not very encouraging. Electric baths as well as static electricity deserve a fair trial in both affections. *Herpes Zoster.*—In the early stage of the eruption the galvanic current, anode to the spine, cathode over the course of the nerve involved, often arrests the pain as well as the eruption. In the post-eruptive neuralgia, which is almost impossible to relieve by any other means, galvanism may be used with expectations of prompt success. The faradic current may also be used, but does not usually act as effectively as galvanism. *Alopecia.*—In the form of baldness known as *alopecia areata* electricity is used with great success. The best method of employing it is by means of the dry faradic brush over the ivory spots. Ranney recommends static sparks very highly. Other forms of alopecia are also benefited by faradization. *Scleroderma and Morphaia.*—Schwimmer reports success in one case of generalized scleroderma after eighteen months' treatment by subaural galvanization. In morphcea localized applications of galvanism have long been regarded as the only treatment that promises success. *Acne.*—Galvanization with anode to the back of the neck and cathode to the seat of eruption often gives the happiest results in chronic, indurated cases. The faradic current is used by many dermatologists with good effects. In torpid cases, with many comedones and few pustules, the dry faradic brush actively applied to the skin is beneficial. Of course, the usual recognized general and local remedies should not be omitted while employing electricity. *Acne Rosacea.*—Central and subaural galvanization are recommended by Beard, E. Remak, and De Watteville. Cases may sometimes yield to this procedure, but where the veins are much dilated, and there is hypertrophy of the skin, a needle connected as cathode is used to puncture all the dilated vessels. The circuit is closed with the anode at an indifferent point—the palm of the hand, for example. In a minute, or less time, with a current of 1 to 2 milliamperes, the blood in the vessel is coagulated or driven out by the evolution of hydrogen gas, and sufficient irritation produced to cause occlusion of the vessel. Multiple galvano-punctures of the hypertrophied skin will also promote atrophy of the latter. This method was first introduced to the notice of the profession by Dr. Hardaway, of St. Louis. Repeated trial has demonstrated its great value in a condition which otherwise is hardly amenable to therapeutic measures. *Ulcers.*—The application of the cathode in form of a metal plate to the surface of the ulcer will stimulate healthy granulation. Where there is too much discharge, or much pain, the anodic application is indicated. Weak currents and long sittings, fifteen to thirty minutes, should be used. The altered nutrition of the granulations is usually promptly manifested. *Parasitic Diseases.*—Against these the electric current itself is of little avail; but advantage may be taken of its cataphoric virtues, as advocated by Dr. Henry J. Reynolds, of Chicago. He applies a solution of mercuric bichloride on the anode to the affected area, and closes the circuit with the cathode at an indifferent point. The penetrating power of the parasiticide is said to be increased by this procedure; *i.e.*, the current *transfers* the bichloride from the surface of the electrode into the hairfollicles and deeper epidermic layers, where it may come in direct contact with the parasite. The observations have been confirmed by others, but the subject requires further and more exact study. *Hypertrichosis.*—The successful employment of electrolysis for the cure of trichiasis f by Dr. Michel, of St. Louis, led Dr. W. A. Hardaway, a distinguished dermatologist of the same Trans. Ninth International Med. Congress, vol. iv. t See *ante,* p. 8OT.

city, to extend the operation to his own special field of practice. The first brilliant successes were obtained in the removal of hairs growing in abnormal situations. Whether the growth be that of a moustache or beard in women, or of growth of hair on the glabella, the tip of the nose, or in the nostrils, electrolysis properly employed will remove the abnormal growth permanently, painlessly, and without leaving any subsequent disfigurement.

Any good constant batter)' will answer the demands of the operation. A current of from J to 2 milliamperes will be necessary.

In addition to a battery in good working order, certain qualifications and appliances are necessary, among which the following are of prime importance:— 1. A plentiful stock of patience.
2. A steady hand. 3. Good eyesight. 4. Proper electrodes. 5. A pair of cilia forceps. 6. A chair with head-rest.

Without the first three natural qualifications mentioned no one should undertake the treatment of a case of hypertrichosis by electrolysis. Defective eyesight may be aided by suitable glasses, but no substitutes can be found for the other two, and a lack of them disqualifies one from properly performing the operation.

The ordinary sponge or cotton-covered disk will answer for the positive electrode. For the negative a needle-holder and fine needle are required.

The holder shown in the cut was devised by Dr. Hardaway, and is made by the A. M. Leslie Company, of St. Louis. It is very convenient. A fine, steel sewing-needle (No. 12) may be used, but flexible needles, made of an alloy of platinum and iridium, are preferable. They are thinner than the finest steel needles, never break, and can be bent into any shape desired. Needle-holders are sometimes made with a key to make and break the circuit, but this is no advantage. The needle is attached to the conducting-wire from the negative pole of the battery.

The forceps should have an easy spring, with flat, lightly serrated jaws, and should not have a catch.

A chair with a firm head-rest must be used. An ordinary cane-seat arm-chair, with adjustable head-rest, answers the purpose as well as a more complicated or expensive oculists' or dentists' chair.

The steps of the operation are as follow:—

The patient is placed before a good light—avoiding direct sunlight, unless modified by frosted glass—and directed to take hold of the handle of the sponge electrode, the sponge, of course, having been previously moistened. The operator then sits a little in front of and to the right of the patient, and takes the needle-electrode in his right hand, holding a pair of tweezers with flat, narrow jaws in his left. The needle is then gently insinuated into a follicle by the side of the hair until the bottom of the follicle is reached. This is manifested by a slight resistance to the onward passage of the needle. The patient is then directed to touch the sponge with the other hand, thus closing the circuit. The current will immediately pass, and the electrolytic action be made manifest by a little frothing around the needle. In some skins also a little wheal will be raised about the follicle. iit from twenty to forty seconds the hair can be extracted with the tweezers without the slightest resistance or pain. If the hair does not come away with perfect ease the papilla has not been destroyed, and the needle should be permitted to remain, and the current to pass a little longer. The circuit is broken by removing the hand from the sponge electrode. This gives less pain than if the circuit is closed and opened with the needle.

If the hairs are very close together they should not all be removed at the same time. The hairs should be picked out here and there, otherwise the points of irritation will be in too close proximity,.and, if sufficiently intense, may produce small areas of sloughing and leave scars. If the operation is properly performed no visible scars should remain.

A sitting may last from fifteen to thirty minutes. Very few operators can extend it beyond the latter time. The sittings may be repeated every other day, or, in cases where time is important, every day.

After the operation a mild astringent lotion may be applied, and the patient should be directed to bathe the surface operated upon several times a day with hot water, for five or ten minutes at a time. This tends to reduce any hyperasmia which may have been caused by the operation.

When the hair-papilla has been thoroughly destroyed the hair cannot be regenerated. In most cases, however, a number of the hairs return, showing that the destruction of the papillae has not been complete. This happens in from 5 to 25 per cent. of the hairs removed, and depends partly upon the skill of the operator and partly upon the direction of the hairs. In some cases the hair shaft in the skin is so twisted that it is almost impossible to strike the papilla. Such hairs often require repeated removal before they are finally destroyed. The greatest success will usually be obtained on the upper lip and chin, while the hairs under the jaw will frequently return again and again, to the great disappointment of both patient and physician. Partial failure should not discourage the operator. Persistence will surely be rewarded by success.

The older the growth of hair, the more satisfactory will be the result. In young persons new hairs continually appear, which sometimes lead the patient to think'that the operation is unsuccessful, and that all the hairs are returning. The fact of the continued growth of the hair should be explained to the patient before beginning the operation. In older persons, where the growth is complete, the new crop consists simply of those hairs which had not been destroyed and which grow ont again. A second removal is followed by still fewer returns, and finally complete success is obtained. In younger individuals this period is longer deferred on account of the above-mentioned outgrowth of new hairs.

Warts, Moles, and Small Fibromata of the Skin.—These growths can be readily removed by electrolysis without leaving disfiguring scars. The process is not painful. The needleholder (Fig. 252) may be employed, but a sharp, steel needle should be used instead of the flexible platinum needle. The flat, lancet-pointed needle sold by the instrument-makers under the name of the "Hagedorn Needle" answers the purpose admirably. The base of the growth is transfixed in various directions, and the current passed for a few minutes each time. The punctured tissues turn pale, and slight frothing occurs around the needle. In most cases the growth, if a wart, mole, or papillary growth, dries into a brownish crust and drops off in the course of a week or ten days, leaving a slightly pigmented spot which soon acquires the natural color of the surrounding skin.

Moles, or pigmented nam of large size, may be effectually removed by this method, leaving little if any disfigurement. Currents of two to six milliamperes may be used.

Milium and Small Wens.—These growths are successfully fully treated by negative galvano-puncture. The centre of the growth is first punctured and the base of the sac touched at a number of points with the needle. Weak currents, one to three milliamperes, are sufficient for the purpose. *Angioma and Teleangiectasis.*—The minute, ampulla-form dilatation of a vessel with radiating branches—the so-called "spider ncevus"—can always be readily destroyed by means of electrolysis. The needle (negative) is plunged into the centre of the dilated vessel, the circuit closed with the anode, and the current ("2 to 3 milliamperes) allowed to pass until the red or brown color has given place to a grayish discoloration. The current is then reversed for a minute or two, making the needle-electrode positive. This insures a firmer clot in the vessel and prevents subsequent haemorrhage. In the course of a week the vessel is usually obliterated and the blemish has disappeared.

Flat, vascular naevi (port-wine mark) and cavernous angiomata of the lip or other portions of the body are amenable to the same course of treatment. Complete success in the removal of these blemishes requires, however, much patience on the part of both physician and patient.

Hypertrophic Scars and Keloid.—Multiple galvano-puncture of the disfiguring scars sometimes remaining after strumous and syphilitic ulcers, or hypertrophic small-pox or vaccination cicatrices, will generally produce much improvement. In true keloid, Dr. W. A. Hardaway, of St. Louis, and Dr. L. Brocq, of Paris, have reported success with the same method, *Epithelioma and Sarcoma.*—In malignant new formations the mild, destructive action of electrolysis has not been much relied upon heretofore, but there is reason to believe that an intelligent use of the method will render resort to the knife or cautery less necessary. Thorough electrolysis of the base of a cancerous or sarcomatous growth can be accomplished if sufficient attention be given to the operation, and the process seems to produce some trophic modification of the tissues which renders a return of the growths less liable to occur than after the use of the knife. This subject deserves a more careful study than has heretofore been given it by surgeons or electro-therapeutists.

When large growths are operated upon it is frequently advisable to use a needle-electrode connected with each pole of the battery and to plunge both needles into the tumor. In this way the resistance to the current is very much diminished and the result is more rapidly obtained. Care must be taken, however, to limit the electrolytic action to the pathological tissue, unless the growth is malignant, when a portion of the normal tissue should also be destroyed to prevent recurrence.

Lupus and Lupus Erythematosus. — Hardaway, who has pointed out so many directions in which the electrolytic method has proven useful in dermatology, was the first to try its effect in lupus erythematosus, making multiple punctures in the morbid tissue. The success was excellent. Like success was obtained in lupus vulgaris. Gartner has employed electrolysis successfully in lupus. He uses a flat metal electrode to produce a superficial slough. This is repeated until the neoplasm is entirely destroyed.

Punctiform galvano-causty with the wire point is also used successfully in lupus.

Elephantiasis Arabum.—Beard and Rockwell give the history of a case of elephantiasis arabum in which great improvement followed the use of the constant current. Since 1877, Professor Silva Araujo, of Rio do Janeiro, has treated upward of four hundred cases with this agent. He studied the effects of electricity upon this morbid condition in connection with Professor Moncorvo, of the same city. The accompanying plates show successive stages of improvement in a case under the treatment as practiced by them. The patient came under treatment in 1879, and was discharged practically cured in 1885. The success in this case and in others reported by Silva Araujo should encourage physicians to persevere in this treatment in suitable cases. The method is as follows: At intervals electrolysis is employed; one, two, or three needles connected with the negative pole are inserted in the densest portion of the hypertrophied tissue, the anode being placed upon the skin near by. The needles are insulated to near their points. Ten-minute sittings are the rule, the needles being withdrawn and re-inserted in another place. During the intervals between the electrolytic sittings daily applications of the constant, followed by the faradic currents, fifteen minutes each, are made. Massage is also practiced, followed by the pure India-rubber bandage to the limb. The massage may be combined with the electricity by using the roller-electrode (Fig. 206).

In the foregoing pages the authors have attempted to give a complete view of the science of electricity and its practical applications in medicine and surgery. They are aware that the work has many shortcomings, but trust that every statement made will bear investigation and criticism. Less attempt has been made to include everything written upon the subject than that nothing untrue should be contained within the covers of the book. If, by its publication,' the means at command to relieve disease or its effects have been extended it will be sufficient reward. In taking leave of their readers, they desire to address to them the final words of Professor Erb: "It will be a source of gratification if your interest in the numerous scientific problems which await solution in this field has been awakened, and it will be a still greater pleasure should you personally contribute by your work to the advancement of Scientific Electrotherapeutics." Elektrothcrapie, 2te aufl., 1S86.

APPENDIX.

Useful Tables And Formulae. *Ohm's Law.* 'Electro-motive force

Current strength =
Resistance.

Electro-motive force = Current strength X resistance.

Electro-motive force *Current Obtainable from any Number of Cells Joined, n in Series, m in Multiple.*

$m n E$
H -j-$m r$

Current = 1 grain (Avoir.)
1 ounce"
1 pound"
1 ton"
=.0648 gramme.
= 28.35 grammes. =.4536 = 1016.' kilos. *Measures of Length.*
1 millimetre (mm.).. =.03937 inch (about *fe* in.)
1 centimetre. =.3937" 1 decimetre... = 3.937 inches. 1 metre. = 39.371" 1 kilometre. = 39371." *Measures of Weight.*
1 milligramme... =.01543 grain (Avoir).
1 centigramme... =.15432"" 1 decigramme,... = 1.5432 grains" 1 gramme. = 15.432 "" 1 kilogramme... = 15432. "" *Resistance of Mixtures of Sulphuric Acid and Water at 22 C. in Terms of Mercury at 0 C. according to Kohlrausch and Nippoldt).*

One ampere flowing during one second decomposes of

Silver, 1.117 milligrammes.
Copper,.....329 milligramme.

The resistances are in ohms, and refer to a length of 100 metres of wire whose diameter is 1 mm.

Change of Resistance of Metals with Change of Temperature. Silver,....0037 to.0041 per ohm (degree C). Copper,....0039 ""
Iron,....0045 ""
German silver,...00028 to.00044""

That is, one ohm of copper wire will become 1.0039 ohms when the temperature is raised one degree centigrade; and three ohms German silver will become 3.00084 to 3.00132 ohms for one-degree-centigrade rise of temperature.

CPSIA information can be obtained at www.ICGtesting.com
Printed in the USA
BVOW01s1048180814

363275BV00021B/805/P